The
GOOD NEWS
About
ESTROGEN

The
GOOD NEWS
About
ESTROGEN

THE TRUTH BEHIND
A POWERHOUSE HORMONE

Uzzi Reiss, M.D.

St. Martin's Press
New York

This book was written for the brave women from all over the world and all walks of life who did not listen to the organized, misleading advice to stop HRT. Their bravery and pursuit of HRT has been paid back with better health, mind, mood, and body.

. . .

In addition, I could not have written this book without the support of my wife of forty-five years, Yael; my daughter, Yfat; daughter-in-law, Llana; and my granddaughters, India, Emerie, and Goldi.

First published in the United States by St. Martin's Press,
an imprint of St. Martin's Publishing Group

www.stmartins.com

Library of Congress Cataloging-in-Publication Data

Names: Reiss, Uzzi, author.
Title: The good news about estrogen : the truth behind a powerhouse hormone / Uzzi Reiss, M.D.
Description: First edition. | New York : St. Martin's Press, 2020. | Includes bibliographical references and index.
Identifiers: LCCN 2019037547 | ISBN 9781250214539 (hardcover) | ISBN 9781250214546 (ebook)
Subjects: LCSH: Estrogen—Therapeutic use. | Menopause—Hormone therapy.
Classification: LCC RG186 .R365 2020 | DDC 618.1/75061—dc23
LC record available at https://lccn.loc.gov/2019037547

Our books may be purchased in bulk for promotional, educational, or business use. Please contact your local bookseller or the Macmillan Corporate and Premium Sales Department at 1-800-221-7945, extension 5442, or by email at MacmillanSpecialMarkets@macmillan.com.

First Edition: March 2020

10 9 8 7 6 5 4 3 2 1

Note to Readers

This book contains my opinions and ideas, which I have formed based on my experience treating women. It is intended to provide helpful general information on the subjects that it addresses. It is not in any way a substitute for the advice of the reader's own physician(s) or other medical professionals based on the reader's own individual conditions, symptoms, or concerns. If the reader needs personal medical, health, dietary, exercise, or other assistance or advice, the reader should consult a competent physician and/or other qualified health care professionals. Both I and my publisher specifically disclaim all responsibility for injury, damage, or loss that the reader may incur as a direct or indirect consequence of following any directions or suggestions given in the book, using any products or services described in the book, or participating in any programs described in the book.

Many of the recommendations and scientific analyses presented in this book are supported by extensive peer-reviewed scientific studies. The bibliography presents much of this supporting research. However, readers can access a complete list of references at my website.

Contents

Contents

Part Two: Estrogen Fallout

Contents

Contents

Introduction

In 2017, the North American Menopause Society announced that "hormone therapy does not need to be routinely discontinued in women older than sixty or sixty-five years and can be considered for continuation beyond sixty-five years. . . . There are not data to support routine discontinuation in women age sixty-five years." This position statement was then supported by the Academy of Women's Health, the American Association of Clinical Endocrinologists, the American Medical Women's Association, and twenty-eight international women's health organizations. Soon after, in that same year, the North American Menopause Society (NAMS) affirmed the "safety and efficacy of hormone therapy for certain conditions and in certain populations of menopausal women." And still later, a study published in late 2017 in the *Journal of the American Medical Association* (*JAMA*) also clarified that using hormone replacement therapy (HRT) for five to seven years was not associated with any risk of disease or mortality. It's now almost three years later, and most women in the United States—indeed, around the world—are still caught up in a misconception about the dangers of estrogen, particularly related to HRT.

At the time of these announcements, the media and medical world paid little attention. Why is this significant? Because the statements supported HRT's safety, dissociating it from increased risk of breast cancer—a major reversal in medical advice. For the fifteen years before 2017, the medical establishment had insisted that any form of HRT was potentially dangerous, which is why so many women avoided hormonal supplementation.

I find this misinformation and misperception about HRT a travesty. Hundreds of millions of women have been missing out on safe, disease-preventing hormone treatment for no good reason.

As an ob-gyn in private practice for over forty years, I have worked with thousands of women, helping them find the healthiest, most effective treatments for their medical problems. As a medical researcher, gynecological specialist, and physician who practices integrative care, I have studied and tested how best to treat women for their individual needs. And the dominant focus of my work has been on revealing to women the power of estrogen, the essential female hormone, to help them defend against disease, offset the effects of aging, and enhance their physical, emotional, and mental well-being. In fact, I believe that estrogen is a superpower for women of any age.

My work with estrogen and other hormones helps women recover from the ill effects of estrogen deficiencies that rob women of their health, vitality, and sometimes even their lives. My integrative approach means that I treat my patients holistically, using a combination of best practices in Western (or allopathic) medicine in addition to nutrition and other functional medicine techniques, so women do not have to wait for disease to occur but rather can take proactive steps to strengthen their body-brain systems as they move through all phases of their lives. It gives me enormous satisfaction to get to know my patients and care for them as they move from adolescence through the early fertility of young adulthood, through perimenopause, and ultimately into menopause. This natural cycle of growth, however, becomes curtailed or disrupted by many culprits: too little estrogen, too much estrogen, and chemicals that have infiltrated your brain and body, disrupting your body's ability to protect itself. In the pages ahead, you will discover a long list of avoidable factors that increase your vulnerability to aging and illness, never mind the effects of hormonal ebbs and flows. Understanding estrogen—its function and interplay with all your other hormones and body systems—is key to boosting your overall health, achieving and maintaining weight loss, increasing your energy, improving your sleep, and gaining inner calm. In short, estrogen and its accompanying hormones can safely turn back the clock and build your capacity to resist the effects of aging.

HRT may not seem like a new solution to fighting the symptoms of perimenopause and menopause. However, my approach is *new*. I treat the whole woman. My patients, from all over the world, come to me because they don't want quick-fix prescriptions or unnecessary surgeries; they want to be in charge of their own health and to make conscious, thoughtful decisions about what feels good and what works. They have come to realize that many conditions, including PMS, osteopenia (low bone density that has not yet developed into osteoporosis), fibroids and endometriosis, and anxiety are preventable once they understand the role of estrogen and other important hormones. Indeed, what distinguishes me and my patients is our mutual trust that, together, they—and you—can achieve optimal hormonal health, which begins with achieving estrogen balance at all times in life.

What also distinguishes me from many other physicians is that I see you—the patient—as a central agent of your own health. In many ways, putting you in control, empowering you with knowledge to make good decisions, is long overdue—women should always be part of their own health care. But I think that we have come to a turning point in medicine: in all specialties it's become clear that patients must be treated as individuals, that a one-size-fits-all basis for diagnosis and treatment is not only ineffective but often dangerous. My biggest breakthrough remains the realization that women need a customized approach to their needs—no one is just like another. They come to me with different life experiences, ethnicities, dietary habits, and exercise histories. Some are aware of genetic markers that may predispose them to certain illnesses; others are not yet aware. I show my patients how to pull together all this vital information so they can become knowledgeable, proactive participants in their own health.

In the pages ahead, you are going to take your own health journey—one that is meant to empower and comfort you. You will learn about how estrogen and other hormones and peptides rule your brain and body; you will learn about what happens emotionally, cognitively, and physically when estrogen begins to dip in midlife. Along the way, you will be prompted to take note of your habits, symptoms, and other health details that will become your hormonal profile, a collection of information that you'll assemble in the health journal entries that you will record as you read this book. You will then be prepared to share your hormonal profile with your physician or health care provider to get what you need. Medicine and science keep moving forward; we have become a drug-dependent culture; my approach is to clean out your medicine cabinet and allow you to rely more on your own body's intelligence to maintain optimal health and well-being—mind and body, which cannot be separated. Again, it's paramount that you take the lead in this process of uncovering what you need to feel and be your best self.

As you will see in the pages of this book, estrogen (as well as other hormones) affects women in different ways for different reasons. Yet every woman is susceptible to the power of estrogen and its ability to optimize her health and protect her from disease and accelerated aging. And no woman is immune to the effects of a decline in estrogen or by the absence of estrogen. Can you be twenty-five and suffering from too little estrogen? Yes. Can you be forty and unaware that you have excessive estrogen because of your exposure to chemicals in your food and cosmetic products? Yes. Can you be in your thirties and catapulted into early menopause because you have been eating a diet high in sugar, starchy carbs, and processed foods and have been exposed to chemicals in your environment? Yes.

Many women who come to see me don't understand the powerful role estrogen plays in their overall health. Many assume that concerns about estrogen are just for women in perimenopause or menopause. I try to dispel these misimpressions. I explain how estrogen is supposed to function in their bodies, how it works with other hormones to coordinate their health. I'll explain this to you, too. Like my patients, you will learn to appreciate that having the proper level of estrogen allows you to avoid many common health problems, including inflammation, thyroid issues, weight gain, the emotional disturbances underlying depression and anxiety, and metabolic disorders such as diabetes and insulin resistance. When your body is out of hormonal balance, you become vulnerable to all sorts of other health issues: endometriosis, fibroids, and other conditions. Perhaps most dramatic, a prolonged estrogen-deficient state can unwittingly and unnecessarily trigger the precursors to heart disease, cognitive decline, and osteoporosis.

Since the publication of two of my previous books, *The Natural Superwoman* (2008) and *Natural Hormone Balance* (2002),

extensive research has been done that shows that bioidentical hormones can be safe and effective in treating a wide range of health
issues and that there are important distinctions between bioidentical hormones and chemicalized (synthetic) hormones. *The Good
News About Estrogen,* my fifth book, covers this new, life-changing
information and offers my comprehensive resource and guide to
hormonal balance. It lays out how you can supplement safely with
bioidentical estrogen and other hormones to improve your overall
health, avoid disease, achieve the best weight for you and your body,
and look and feel so much better. I want you to find in these pages
everything you need to know about the powerful role of estrogen
in your health—whatever your age. After forty years of working
on the front lines of women's health, I believe strongly that every
woman—not just those who are my patients—has the right to make
her own choices about her health. As a physician, I want to expose
the dangerous side effects that some prescription medications can
cause, the still-rising costs of these pharmaceutical products, and
the resulting hospitalizations that can create further problems.

Wouldn't you like to learn how taking a simple supplement of
estrogen and/or progesterone can enhance your brain, your body,
and your beauty?

In *The Good News About Estrogen,* I give you the information
you need—from a point of view you can trust—to protect your life
so that you can have the best chance of feeling vibrant, energetic,
and youthful now and into the future.

You will learn how

- a simple daily dose of a bioidentical transdermal cream or
  gel can protect you against heart disease
- this same daily dose can also protect you against osteoporosis and improve your sleep, anxiety, and mood
- the link between estrogen and memory works and how

estrogen in its bioidentical form can improve your brain power

- estrogen can enhance your skin's elasticity and give you tighter, more vital-looking skin
- you can continue to maintain a healthy sexual life and enjoy all that sex can bring

The Good News About Estrogen demystifies estrogen and tells you the truth about its importance in your body and mind, your health, and your life. You will also learn the "real deal" about the safety of mammograms and the dangers of overdiagnosis of breast cancer. Did you know, for instance, that many of the "tumors" caught by mammograms are benign? I understand this sounds controversial. Every woman I have ever encountered is terrified of developing breast cancer. But the truth is that the way most health care practitioners think about and treat women's bodies is completely outdated. They do not have access to current research and practices and in some cases are using inaccurate, incomplete methods of diagnosis and treatment. They could be using less invasive approaches that are more holistic with fewer negative side effects and consequences. And, most alarmingly, they are not giving women the information they need *ahead of time* to prevent many conditions.

In this book, you have a concise, thorough guide to figure out what your body needs, what supplements and nutrients you can benefit from, and what other lifestyle practices will support your overall hormonal health. I will share with you how women in my practice have made small but powerful changes to the way they eat, sleep, and exercise (as little as fifteen minutes a day) to reset their bodies and boost their hormonal balance and how you can make important changes, too. Yes, you will learn how to feel and look better. You can regain energy, focus, and a sense of optimism—all of which tend to dwindle with the loss of estrogen. But even more important, you will learn methods that can help you protect yourself against breast cancer, heart disease, and cognitive decline.

Again, the medical information and recommendations given here are informed by hundreds of peer-reviewed, replicated studies that support both the safety and efficacy of taking, in a dose appropriate for you, bioidentical estrogen and other hormones. (For a thorough list of the most important references, please see the bibliography at the back of the book; you can also access a complete bibliography on my website, www.uzzireissmd.com). Of course, you should always work with your physician to determine whether and how to implement any information in these pages in a manner that is safe and effective for you as an individual.

The Good News About Estrogen is actually much more than a guide to hormonal health. It's a crucial, lifesaving challenge that asks you to make a profound change in how you think about your own vitality and about estrogen: I want you to question the pervasive misinformation that now stokes so many women's fear of estrogen. I want you to accept estrogen for the wonderful, enlivening powerhouse hormone it is.

I care deeply about empowering you, protecting your health, and giving you the accurate information you need. I offer information and advice that I would give to treat my wife, my daughter, my daughter-in-law, and my three granddaughters. I don't want you to sit on the sidelines of life, feeling low, tired, and depressed, waiting for an inevitable decline in your health. Getting proper treatment with estrogen can help many women feel good again. Please join me in the following pages to learn how.

Part One

. . . .

Estrogen: Your Brain and Body's Conductor

1

What Estrogen Does for
Your Body and Brain

n this chapter, I share with you specific information about how estrogen functions in your body and brain, so that you can become aware of how hormones are supposed to function in your body. Your hormonal system represents the pinnacle of how your body and brain work together. I like to think of this interaction as a symphony, with estrogen as lead conductor. It's estrogen's role to bring together all the other hormones and help them interact to ensure that you are healthy.

As you think about your own situation, and whether or not you feel ready to benefit from bioidentical hormone replacement therapy (HRT), it's important to understand how estrogen is meant to function—both throughout your monthly cycle and over your lifetime so that you can fully appreciate and become more aware of the changes—subtle and not so subtle—that continue to occur.

Your Monthly Cycle

After the onset of puberty and before menopause, your estrogen levels fluctuate over the course of every month. A "typical" monthly cycle lasts approximately 28 days, though some women experience a brief 24-day cycle and others can have a 35-day cycle. A monthly cycle that is shorter or longer than 28 days is no less "normal" than a cycle that adheres precisely to a four-week schedule. What's normal for you . . . may not be normal for another woman.

Week 1

The first day of menstruation is day 1 of your monthly cycle. This is the day the body begins its preparations to conceive in the upcoming month. Typically, menstruation lasts 5–7 days. During the first few days of menstruation, estrogen levels are very low, which is the main cause of the tiredness, lack of energy, low mood, trouble sleeping, cramping, and other symptoms that many women experience. By day 5 or so, estrogen levels begin to rise, and many women feel energized, centered, and even-keeled. That week after you've completed your period, when you feel as though you're firing on all cylinders—rested, full of energy, enjoying the way you look and feel—you have estrogen to thank for that. This estrogen cycle is part of a network of brain–body signals that drive the body's quest for reproduction.

Week 2

During days 7–14 of your monthly cycle, estrogen levels rise significantly. For many women, this week feels like a gift—they are energetic and productive. You may feel tremendously capable, sexy and sexually motivated, attractive and centered. During this week, estrogen is climbing toward its peak level, which comes just before ovulation. This rise in estrogen makes your skin look pretty, dewy, and clear. Women tend to feel most powerful and womanly during this phase of their cycle. The reason for this is no mystery: this is nature's way of encouraging conception.

While you are feeling all the positive, vibrant, sexy effects of rising estrogen, that same estrogen surge is helping prepare your body to conceive. Estrogen increases production of cervical mucus, which will corral sperm that have entered the vagina and pull them through the cervix toward an egg waiting to be fertilized. Estrogen also promotes the thickening of the uterus's lining, where an embryo will implant after the biologically hoped-for fertilization occurs.

Right before ovulation, estrogen levels drop briefly and precipitously, which is accompanied by a surge of testosterone. With this increase in testosterone, you might feel a more intense, urgent desire for sex than you do under the influence of the sensuality-promoting estrogen. On the cusp of ovulation, this is the body's final push toward reaching its goal of conception.

Week 3

After that sharp drop just before ovulation, estrogen levels begin to rise again gradually during days 14–21 of a woman's cycle, though not to the levels they reached just prior to ovulation. After having spent two weeks preparing to conceive, your body now functions as if it were pregnant. This can mean a continuation of the "feel-good" times of the pre-ovulation week, albeit slightly muted and without the same intensity of sexual energy. Immediately upon ovulation, the body began producing greater amounts of progesterone, which has a mood-balancing, calming effect. As women age, the estrogen rebound that occurs after ovulation often changes. The pre-ovulation drop in estrogen becomes steeper and estrogen levels fall further than when women were younger. The subsequent rise in estrogen also takes longer to occur, as many as several days or a week. Women in their thirties and forties may come to experience this week of their cycle very differently than they did when they were younger, with increasing symptoms of estrogen decline and deficiency.

Week 4

The week before menstruation, a woman's body recognizes it is not pregnant. (Unless, of course, you are.) This biological moment of truth triggers estrogen to decline, leading to many of the symptoms associated with PMS: trouble sleeping, fatigue, mood swings, feelings of depression, forgetfulness, headaches. Progesterone, while still being produced by the ovaries, is also on the decline during this week, causing bloating, feelings of anxiousness, and breast fullness and tenderness. Testosterone levels rise during this premenstrual week, leading to feelings of irritability, as well as oily skin.

As women age, the decline in estrogen—as well as accompanying changes to levels of progesterone and testosterone—may begin earlier and earlier, cutting into the third week of the monthly cycle. The estrogen drop that ushers in the uncomfortable, painful, sometimes debilitating symptoms of estrogen deficiency and PMS can start as early as day 15 of a woman's cycle, very shortly after ovulation itself. Estrogen reaches its lowest level just before a woman's menstrual flow, and a new monthly cycle begins.

If progesterone drops, you spot before your period, and if progesterone falls too soon, you don't reach the usual 28th day of a normal cycle and don't bleed at all.

The Subtypes of Estrogen

Estrogen is often discussed as though it were a single hormone. In fact, there are several estrogens, including one estrogen compound—esterol, or E4—that is made only during pregnancy. The three most important estrogen compounds that all women's bodies produce are estradiol (E2), estrone (E1), and estriol (E3). The ovaries, the primary place of estrogen production in the body, make these three different versions of the hormone.

Estradiol (E2)—The most potent and efficient of the estrogens, estradiol is responsible for many of the protective health benefits for which estrogen is known. With receptors on every cell in your body, estradiol affects most of your body's systems—from reproduction to digestion and everything in between.

Estrone (E1)—A weaker version of estrogen, estrone is produced by the ovaries and liver before menopause; after menopause, estrone is produced by your fat cells. It is thought to help retain bone strength.

Estriol (E3)—This estrogen compound is markedly weaker than both estradiol and estrone. Ninety-nine percent weaker than E2, estriol is a gentle version of estrogen that plays a critical role in balancing the other estrogens. It mainly functions during pregnancy (when it increases a thousandfold), and is often an indication of the health of a pregnancy. When it comes to HRT, estriol is very important to balancing the way the other estrogens work. Most significant among its functions is that estriol protects against breast cancer. It also supports vaginal health, maintaining lubrication, encouraging production of good bacteria (which means fewer vaginal and urinary infections), and restoring the tissues of the vaginal wall. Estriol helps skin remain youthful, full, and elastic, and it reduces inflammation.

Each of these estrogen compounds produced by the body has its own role in creating health, sexual function, and mental and emotional well-being. Working in collaboration, estrogens protect cardiovascular health, regulate appetite and weight, boost energy, keep the brain and bones healthy and strong, balance mood, and protect against depression and anxiety. Together, these three estrogens keep you feeling like your best self: healthy, capable, energized, and focused. So my question to you is this: why not live a long life enjoying their many benefits?

The Life Cycle of Estrogen

Puberty

Estrogen drives much of the development from girlhood to womanhood—it fosters breast development, inaugurates and supports reproductive capabilities, and facilitates the gravitation of fat to a girl's hips, legs, and breasts. Prepubescent girls have consistently low levels of estrogen in their bodies. At the onset of puberty, the ovaries begin to ramp up estrogen production. It's at this time that estrogen—along with progesterone and testosterone—begins to rise and to fluctuate significantly. Estrogen is the driving force behind the development of a maturing girl's curves, the onset of her menses and her ability to conceive, and the dawning of her sexuality. Estrogen also contributes to distinct changes to her emotional and psychological life and experiences, both as an individual and in her relationships with others. As you read the stories of my patients, you will come to recognize the connections between estrogen and a woman's sense of self.

As puberty progresses, estrogen and other hormones often behave erratically, working to come into balance. Irregular menstrual cycles, cramping, mood swings, and other symptoms associated with PMS are commonly experienced among girls moving through puberty.

The typical age of puberty has lowered significantly over the past twenty years. While it was once common for puberty to begin somewhere in mid-adolescence, around the ages of 14–17, today the onset of puberty happens much earlier, with an average age of menarche, the beginning of menstruation, between ages 11–13. The reasons behind this shift are complicated. A significant root cause for early puberty is exposure to the chemicals in household products, including cosmetics and hygiene products. These chemicals mimic estrogen and give a young girl's body and hormonal system the false impression that she has a lot of estrogen, and so the body responds by beginning puberty earlier than it would if she did not have daily exposure to chemicals.

Food also plays a role in the early onset of puberty. Researchers believe that girls who eat a diet high in nonorganic or processed/packaged foods high in fat and sugar mature earlier than did girls in the past. In addition, some researchers believe that early menarche is tied to fat mass: the heavier the girl, the more likely she will start her period at a younger age. And many girls are heavier today than in previous generations.

Getting your period early in life is not necessarily a health concern. However, it is a signal that a girl's body is responding to environmental triggers that may not be good for her. (See chapters 2 and 10 on how to avoid these triggers and protect a young woman's reproductive health.)

Young Adulthood

Estrogen levels, rising throughout puberty, typically reach their peak in your midtwenties. This peak is also the time when women generally are most fertile. Often, the irregularity of estrogen's monthly rise and fall—as well as the rise and fall of other hormones, including testosterone and progesterone—evens out by young adulthood. During their twenties and early thirties, women generally have consistent month-to-month estrogen fluctuations and predictable symptoms from the normal rise and fall of estrogen and other hormones. Yet for many women today, biological fertility does not align easily with social, professional, and relationship pressures. In other words, young women have many competing goals during this fertile period.

Perimenopause

Perimenopause is the transition from the hormonal routine of a woman's reproductive years to menopause. Perimenopause typically begins five to ten years before menopause, often in a woman's early forties. Over the past two decades, clinicians and researchers, including me, have seen more women entering perimenopause earlier than was typical in previous generations. It is no longer unusual for women to enter perimenopause in their thirties, and for women in their late twenties to have estrogen deficiencies. This shift seems primarily due to both xenoestrogens and the widespread prescription and use of birth control pills, which interrupt the natural production of estrogen and are prescribed for reasons other than preventing pregnancy. For instance, the Pill is used to treat acne, anxiety, and sometimes even ADHD.

Perimenopause can be a time of great hormonal irregularity. Estrogen levels are declining overall—but not in a linear, even fashion. During perimenopause, estrogen seesaws up and down, fluctuating dramatically and erratically, without the same pattern of fluctuation that once occurred in younger years. The result? Unpredictable, variable monthly menstruation cycles, with irregular periods that change in their duration and in the amount of bleeding a woman experiences from one month to the next.

Women also experience symptoms of pronounced estrogen deficiency, including night sweats and hot flashes, mood swings, depleted energy, headaches, weight gain, and diminished interest in sex. I find that blood tests to measure estrogen levels as a clinical yardstick for menopause are useful, but to a limited degree. Women who fall in the wide range of "normal" estrogen levels indicated by blood tests can be firmly within perimenopause, as evidenced by their symptoms. And these symptoms can increase in severity. As you will see in chapter 4, it's important to cue into any changes in your cycle and become familiar with signs of deficiency.

Progesterone in Perimenopause and Menopause

While estrogen rises and decreases dramatically even as it gradually declines over your lifetime, progesterone diminishes steadily starting in the early thirties, before declining markedly around age thirty-five. In previous generations, it was uncommon to enter menopause before fifty-five years old, but women today can enter menopause as young as thirty-eight or forty. Without a natural progesterone supply, you lose the balancing effect that progesterone provides to estrogen, as well as the protections against heart disease, breast cancer, cognitive decline, and other conditions. You will learn more about progesterone and its role in your overall hormonal health on page 46.

Menopause

What is menopause? Is it the absence of a period? Is it a check-list of symptoms—night sweats, hot flashes, mood swings, weight gain? I regard menopause as a persistent state of estrogen deficiency. The cessation of menstruation and the range of symptoms that we associate with menopause are consequences of this underlying lack of estrogen.

Looking at menopause this way—as a deficiency of estrogen—you can see that menopause isn't something that ends. Your hormonal life changes when menopause begins, but there is no end point at which you will be beyond estrogen deficiency. For this reason, I never talk about patients being "postmenopausal." Women experience menopause and declining estrogen differently. Overall, early menopause involves larger and more frequent fluctuations and stronger reactions to estrogen deprivation, with more pronounced symptoms. As menopause progresses, some outward symptoms may quiet and recede—but the gradual dwindling of estrogen continues.

Let's take a look at the phases of menopause and how estrogen behaves during each phase. It's important to identify where you are in menopause when you're working with your physician to design a bioidentical hormone replacement regimen that fits your individual needs. And remember, you experience the phases of estrogen in your own way, depending on your own particular hormonal identity. Many physicians refuse to prescribe estrogen until complete menopause; this is a mistake, causing many women to suffer unnecessarily for years. (See chapter 6 to take steps to understand your individual hormonal profile.) A significant factor in how you become menopausal is how much estrogen your body has produced throughout the course of your life since puberty. Other factors include how regular or irregular your cycle has been, if you experienced PMS, and how much you bled or didn't bleed. Don't be alarmed if your experience doesn't exactly match the following, somewhat typical, descriptions. Variations are natural.

EARLY MENOPAUSE

Also known as early-onset menopause, this phase comprises approximately the first three years of menopause. By this point, women have stopped menstruating. Estrogen levels are still capable of frequent and strong fluctuations, but these rises and falls are less dramatic than they were during perimenopause. Because estrogen levels overall have declined significantly in early menopause, the symptoms of estrogen deficiency can be severe.

MID-MENOPAUSE

The next five years of menopause are considered mid-menopause. At this point, the body has been producing estrogen levels that are for the most part consistently low, with occasional fluctuations. Many women during mid-menopause experience fewer hot flashes and night sweats, symptoms associated with estrogen deficiency. This quieting of symptoms can lead women to believe they have moved beyond menopause, which doesn't happen. In mid-menopause, women continue to experience the effects of estrogen deficiency, even as their bodies and minds make adjustments to cope with the symptoms. But their underlying estrogen deprivation remains, until or unless they are supplementing with bioidentical estrogen.

LATE MENOPAUSE

Most women over the age of fifty-eight have entered the late phase of menopause, which on average has been going on for at least ten years. Estrogen levels in this phase of menopause are low but constant, with virtually no fluctuation. Late menopause is the "phase" in which women will remain for the rest of their lives. Late menopause—or any stage of menopause—should not be equated with giving up or giving in to the effects of estrogen deficiency. This need not be a time for settling or learning to live with less—less energy, less sex, less mental and intellectual sharpness, less joy and fulfillment. Last year, Irene, a seventy-five-year-old patient of mine who had not been sexually active for twenty years, began to enjoy a new romance. She became sexually active with her new partner and even experienced an orgasm. The ability of the vagina lining to become lubricated can always be improved with HRT and supplements. Unfortunately, men's plumbing issues—whether related to incontinence or sexual functioning—can't be restored, but women are lucky!

Up until around age fifty-eight—most women after fifty-eight can no longer produce estrogen—adult women who have low estrogen can benefit from bioidentical estrogen, tailored to meet their individual hormonal needs. This is true for young women, for women in the throes of perimenopausal estrogen decline, and for women who have been in menopause for many years. As I tell my patients, what's good for women at twenty is still good for them at seventy! If you think you might be estrogen deficient, keep in mind that getting such HRT can help bone to regrow and help improve skin health. Receiving bioidentical HRT can also wake up the vagina, which will enhance your ability to experience sexual pleasure.

The Problems with Excessive Estrogen

Though excess estrogen rarely occurs on its own, in today's world, our bodies are assaulted by an array of toxic chemicals that permeate our environment and appear in the food we eat, the water we drink, the air we breathe, and the products we use in our homes and workplaces. Many chemicals, once inside the body, mimic the functions and effects of estrogen and raise risks of developing breast cancer and other cancers. Known as xenoestrogens, these chemicals affect girls and even babies in the womb, and this early-in-life exposure to toxins and chemicals increases the risk of breast cancer throughout their lifetime. These estrogenic chemicals also wreak havoc on women's bodies. In addition, excess estrogen is frequently and inaccurately used by practitioners as a marker to determine how much estrogen a woman needs; often resulting in women receiving a sub-optimal amount.

Xenoestrogens are found in numerous products, from shampoo and deodorant to canned goods and plastic containers. Xenoestrogens wreak havoc with natural hormone levels, trigger inflammation throughout the body, damage genes, and distort gene function—all of which also raises the risk for cancers. Some of the chemicals most abundantly present in the environment that are associated with breast cancer risk include the following:

Dioxins. Dioxins are a group of highly toxic chemicals that act as xenoestrogens and specifically affect hormonal health. By-products of a wide range of manufacturing processes, including smelting, chlorine bleaching of paper pulp, and the manufacturing of some herbicides and pesticides, dioxins are released into the environment, with the highest levels of these compounds found in some soils, sediments, and food, especially nonorganic dairy products, meat, fish, and shellfish. **They are among the "dirty dozen," a list of the most dangerous and widespread persistent organic pollutants, or POPs, we are unwittingly exposed to through the foods we eat.** Dioxins have long been identified as a serious health hazard, and efforts to reduce their levels in food and at large have been under way for years. Federal restrictions on dioxin production limit the amount of the chemical that can be generated, and screenings exist for dioxin levels in food, both within the United States and outside it. But dioxins, like other POPs, don't just disappear—they remain lodged in the cells and tissues of plants and animals, in the water, and in the air. Because of so many years of accumulated dioxins, exposure to this group of toxins remains widespread and, to a real degree, unavoidable.

- Dioxin is a xenoestrogen; it functions like estrogen in the body, disrupting hormone balance and raising risks for cancer.
- Dioxin raises risks for cancers in the general population.
- Dioxin elevates the risk for breast cancer and other cancers.
- Dioxin exposure in utero affects that unborn child's risk for breast cancer throughout her lifetime.
- Dioxin exposure can cause reproductive problems and fertility issues.
- Dioxin damages the immune system.
- Dioxin exposure is especially harmful in people who eat high-fat diets.

BPA (bisphenol A). BPA is found in plastics and epoxy resins used to coat metal, including cans for food. Humans are widely exposed to BPA in food, in water and air, and through everyday products found at home and work. This toxin is also found in many consumer plastics, including cans for food, plastic food storage bags, plastic utensils for eating and drinking, water bottles, other plastic containers such as CD or DVD cases, and electronic equipment. Work has been done in recent years to remove BPA from consumer products, and it's common now to see plastics and cans used for consumer products, including food products and products for children and babies, labeled BPA-free. We must ask ourselves, however, whether what's being used in place of BPA is truly safer (see below on BBPs). Like other persistent organic pollutants, BPA cannot simply be removed from circulation; this dangerous xenoestrogen remains throughout the environment—in our water supplies and in our food chain.

- BPA is a xenoestrogen, and exposure to this toxin—especially during youth—raises risks for breast cancer and other cancers.
- BPA triggers changes to normal cell growth and alters apoptosis (orderly cell death), increasing cancer risk.
- BPA is linked to cardiovascular problems in men and women.
- BPA elevates risks for cancers, diabetes, cognitive dysfunction, and asthma.

BBP (benzyl butyl phthalate). This chemical, used in plastics manufacturing, is another xenoestrogen to which humans are broadly exposed. Significantly disruptive not only to estrogen but also to testosterone, BBP and other phthalates are found in vinyl, PVC, and plastics used in commercial and consumer products. Exposure to BBP comes through food and water sources, as well as through direct contact with plastics. BBP exposure in utero is linked to elevated lifetime breast cancer risk. Exposure during a woman's lifetime also raises her risk.

- BBP spurs the growth of breast cancer cells.
- Exposure to BBP in utero leads to changes in gene expression that make a woman more vulnerable to breast cancer (and other cancers) throughout her lifetime.
- BBP increases incidence of polycystic ovary syndrome (PCOS)
- BBP contributes to fertility problems in men and women.
- BBP is linked to developmental delays in children.
- BBP may contribute to obesity.
- BBP triggers, aggravates, and causes asthma.

DDT (dichlorodiphenyltricholoroethane). Another of the dirty dozen POPs, DDT is a pesticide that was widely used in commercial and industrial agriculture before its ban in the United States in 1972. But it persists in the environment and is still used in other parts of the world, primarily to kill mosquitoes that spread disease.

- DDT exposure at a young age dramatically increases a woman's risk for breast cancer throughout her lifetime.
- Maternal exposure to DDT is highly predictive of daughters' breast cancer, raising this next generation's breast cancer risk by 370 percent.
- DDT may contribute to other cancers.
- DDT contributes to fertility and reproductive problems.
- DDT can damage the nervous system.

PAH (polycyclic aromatic hydrocarbons). PAH are chemicals produced from burning fossil fuels and the burning of other substances, including wood, garbage, and tobacco. Cigarette smoke contains high levels of PAH. PAH are absorbed by the human body through air, food, and water. Many PAH are xenoestrogens.

- Early-in-life exposure to PAH elevates risk of breast cancer throughout a woman's lifetime.
- A woman's PAH exposure at the time of her first pregnancy may affect her risk of breast cancer later in life, after she has transitioned to menopause.
- PAH elevate risks for other cancers in women and in men.
- PAH contribute to disorders and diseases of lungs, gastrointestinal system, kidneys, and skin.

Ethanol. Ethanol is touted as a "green" alternative to gasoline and is often used as an additive to it. Scientists have found that ethanol and its by-products create ground-level ozone pollution, adding toxicity to our air and water. Exposure to ethanol raises risks for breast cancer.

Aluminum. This abundant metal is used widely in commercial, industrial, and consumer activities, production, and products. Aluminum is also a common ingredient in personal care products, including deodorants, makeup, toothpaste, and sunscreen, as well as in medications such as antacids and some aspirins. Aluminum is sometimes used as an additive to food.

A hormone- and estrogen-disrupting metal, aluminum exposure is linked to

- Neurodegenerative disease, including Alzheimer's disease
- Nervous system damage
- Alterations to DNA
- Cancers, including breast cancer

Cadmium. This heavy metal is created as a by-product of industrial production and the burning of fossil fuels. It is also released in tobacco smoke. Cadmium is a widespread contaminant in soil and water and so makes its way into our food. Cadmium is used in chemical fertilizers, chemical dyes, plastics, and batteries. A hormone disruptor, cadmium exposure results in imbalance to estrogen and overall hormone balance.

- Chronic exposure to cadmium has been shown to elevate breast cancer risk.
- Cadmium exposure can be damaging to kidneys and kidney function.
- Exposure to cadmium can cause lung disease.
- Cadmium is associated with cardiovascular disease risk.
- Cadmium contributes to developmental defects.

Endocrine-disrupting chemicals can be found anywhere in your home—from the laundry room and kitchen to the bathroom, living room, and bedroom. Essentially, any piece of furniture, rug or carpet, cosmetic, or cleaning product can contain a dangerous chemical. Absorbed into the body through air, water, and food, as well as direct contact with chemicals and the products they generate, environmental toxins gather and lodge in fatty tissues, like the tissue of the breast. A toxic environment poses profound health hazards that our preindustrial ancestors did not face. Science and medicine have barely begun to understand these modern problems, and of the tens of thousands of chemicals found in consumer and industrial products, very few have been subjected to rigorous scientific study. We know very little about the chemical toxins that surround us, but one thing we do know: cancer rates have soared alongside the industrial and technological development of the last century. We also know that you can take proactive steps to protect yourself and your family. First, make it a habit to look at the labels of all household, cosmetic, and personal health products you consider purchasing. Many times, the chemicals or their derivatives are identified. Safe products are typically labeled as such with language such as "Non-GMO" or "No parabens or other harmful chemicals." In my experience, the Environmental Working Group (EWG) is a reliable source for learning more about individual chemicals as well as safer products you can use on your body and in your home.

The youngest and the eldest among us are more vulnerable to these chemicals because their immune systems are not as strong or protective. In some cases, metals, for instance, can be removed from the body. In other cases, you can take steps to "detoxify" your body and lessen or remove the chemicals that have accumulated. A very first step is to reduce exposure; then the body will naturally and automatically use its own detox strategies to get rid of foreign agents—through sweat, excretion, and sleep.

Environmental Hazards

Chemical toxins elevate the risk for breast and other cancers through several different pathways:

Oxidative stress. The process of oxidative stress in the body generates free radicals. These are molecules broken away from whole, stable cells that damage tissues and healthy cells and promote the initial development and growth of cancer cells.

Inflammation. Environmental toxins can trigger unhealthy levels of inflammation in the body. The presence of inflammation promotes aromatization—the conversion of testosterone to estrogen in the breast, which elevates risk for breast cancer. Inflammation increases the aggressiveness of breast cancer, and the likelihood of metastasis, as well as the risks for other cancers and disease.

Damage to DNA and genetic function. Many of the chemicals we are exposed to are genotoxic, which means they directly affect genes and DNA. The accumulation of chemicals in breast tissue and other tissues of the body causes damage to genes and to their ideal, intended function and expression. Mutations and alterations to normal gene structure and function lead to disease, including breast cancer.

Hormone disruption. Many environmental chemicals and toxins disrupt endocrine function, upending the delicate balance of hormones in the body. A great many of the most toxic and widespread chemicals found in our environment are xenoestrogens, chemicals that can both mimic and disrupt estrogen when absorbed into the body, leading to estrogen imbalance and elevating risks for breast cancer, metabolic disorders, cardiovascular problems, cognitive decline, and a broad range of illness and disease.

Women Vary

Just as a woman's estrogen levels fluctuate throughout each month and over the course of her lifetime, every woman's estrogen "identity" is different—both in the patterns of estrogen's rise and fall and in how much estrogen her body naturally produces. Consider the situation of fifty-two-year-old fraternal twin sisters whom I treat. Mary, a mother of three teenage daughters, is five foot five and athletic and has thick brown and gray hair. She has fairly high muscle mass, experiences severe PMS, and bleeds heavily and regularly every month. Her sister Megan is five foot four, slightly built, and weighs twenty pounds less than her sister. Megan no longer gets her period (she went into menopause at forty-nine) and has never given birth.

Although the two women resemble each other, they have markedly different hormonal identities, due to many factors, most important of which are their differing levels of estrogen, progesterone, and testosterone. Mary has high levels of testosterone, very low levels of progesterone, and uneven estrogen levels—in other words, they vary throughout the month. Megan is low in all three hormones, in part because she never got pregnant and has a slight build. (It's also important to note that testosterone levels are often inaccurate, as this hormone can exist intra-cellularly as well.)

Although Mary and Megan share a tremendous amount of DNA and were raised in the same household, their life experiences (pregnancy versus no pregnancy) set them apart, as do their body types. The fact that Megan is in menopause and Mary is not (she is in perimenopause, four to eight years prior to the cessation of menstruation) is probably the biggest marker setting the twins' health profiles apart. Megan's hormonal levels are lower than those of her sister, who is still menstruating. Neither woman is less or more healthy than the other—they just need different amounts and combinations of hormonal supplements.

Women's bodies naturally produce different levels of estrogen. Some women naturally produce high levels of estrogen, while others produce barely a sufficient amount to enable fertility. Women who have high levels of estrogen are typically short in stature, full breasted, and curvy. Women who naturally produce less estrogen tend to be tall, thin, and small breasted. Estrogen speeds up development and maturation, which includes helping bones to "close," which in turn signals the body to stop growing. The great majority of women fall somewhere in between these highest and lowest estrogen producers. However, how consistently a woman produces estrogen over the course of her life, especially during her main reproductive years, reflects and predicts her body's ability to protect itself from degeneration. In general, women who make sufficient estrogen, live a healthy lifestyle, and stay away from environmental toxins that interfere with hormonal balance will be in a better position to protect their overall health and well-being.

So how do you know what is a sufficient amount of estrogen for your health? It's very difficult to define a "normal" hormone level for any one woman, because what is a so-called normal or healthy amount for one woman is not right for another. Patients and doctors all need to be aware of this essential variation so that, once you begin a regimen, you can continue to talk to your physician about your symptoms—which ones have resolved and which are persistent—and have the physician adjust your dose to the amount that works best for you. For instance, many doctors insist that a level of 50 picograms (pg/ML) is "enough," despite the variation in individuals' blood hormone levels. Often this is the amount delivered by an estrogen patch, which is minimally efficient and effective.

However, in my experience 50 pg/ML is not at all sufficient for most women. Doctors used to be mainly concerned about night sweats, which is how they originally came up with 50 pg/ML as a sufficient level. However, if a woman has always shown a blood level over 200 pg/ML, receiving only 50 pg/ML once she is in menopause will not be nearly sufficient to solve her mood, sleep, or fatigue issues or let her feel like herself again. All these numbers and measurements will make more sense after you read the successive chapters and begin to assemble your own hormonal profile.

Even though each woman experiences the ebb and flow of estrogen differently, there are common symptoms that indicate when you are in a state of high estrogen or low estrogen. Learning to recognize these symptoms can help you better weather hormonal shifts and help you anticipate and manage symptoms amid your daily life. You can develop a sense of what to expect physically, mentally, and emotionally rather than feeling broadsided by fatigue, irritability, or memory problems. Understanding when and why these and other symptoms occur makes them much easier to deal with—and allows you to make decisions about whether, and when, to use supplemental estrogen and other hormones.

There is no more valuable information than your understanding and awareness of your own body—how you feel, under what conditions you function at your best, and how you respond to changes in your estrogen levels. These are the truest guides to health and wellness as you age. The most important insights—about estrogen, and more broadly about hormone balance—can't be read on a chart or gleaned from a lab result. They come from you, your deep capacity for self-awareness, and your thoughtful attention to your mental and physical feelings.

Clearing the Air: The Difference Between Chemical and Bioidentical Hormones

For too long, bioidentical hormones—estrogen and others—have been lumped together with chemicalized (or synthetic) hormones and have been regarded as essentially the same, with the same risks and benefits. However, bioidentical hormones have far fewer risks than synthetics do. By and large, physicians recommending HRT default to prescribing chemicalized estrogen and progesterone supplements because they are easier to access, are more often covered by insurance, and remain part of our culture's outsize trust in big pharma. I believe that the benefits of using bioidentical hormones far outweigh their downsides—namely, inconvenience, since obtaining them requires that you see a health practitioner who works individually with a compounding pharmacy. Of course, this decision is up to you—at the end of the day, I'd prefer that you receive some supplementation to none.

All bioidentical hormones are created through an enzymatic process that takes specific molecules in plants, such as organic yams and soy, and makes the hormone identical in structure to the hormones created by the human body. Down to the molecule, bioidentical estrogen is the same as human estrogen. For this reason, I believe that bioidentical estrogen is a safer, effective way to replace diminishing estrogen levels as you age and move through perimenopause and menopause.

On the other hand, chemicalized estrogen is the synthetic or chemicalized estrogen in medications, such as Premarin and Provera, often prescribed by physicians who do not use bioidenticals. Pharmaceutical corporations generate the vast majority of estrogen that women use in hormone replacement therapy. The estrogens made by pharmaceutical manufacturers from animal and plant sources are synthesized to their own proprietary, patented versions of estrogen—which, of course, is the key to their profitability. Many chemicalized estrogen substitutes are what's known as conjugated equine estrogens, or CEEs. To my knowledge, there is no scientific basis for preferring estrogen supplements for women that are created from horse urine. Horse urine contains several different estrogens (twelve, to be exact), and all but one are biochemically distinct from a human female's estrogen. Horse urine is used, it appears, out of ease and economy. Horses have long gestation periods and large bladders, and they can be constantly catheterized to draw urine that winds up in medication used by millions of women each year. Most women have no idea where their estrogen comes from or what animals go through for them to get it. I believe that these CEEs are inferior estrogen that may actually cause harm to the women they purport to help.

Other, newer forms of chemicalized estrogen are synthesized from plants, primarily from soy. That might sound like a step in the right direction, but the final estrogen compounds made from these plant sources are synthesized to be biochemical matches to the CEEs of earlier generations, not to a woman's own estrogen. This approach may protect the proprietary nature of the product, but it does nothing advantageous for women who need estrogen that matches their own. Nevertheless, these plant-derived estrogens are marketed as "natural," despite the fact that they're closer biochemically to the natural estrogen of a horse than that of a woman.

Chemicalized estrogens often use a version of only one of the three estrogen compounds—estradiol, E2, the strongest of the estrogens found naturally in women. Estradiol delivers powerful benefits, but those benefits are maximized—and its risks minimized—when E2 exists in balance with estriol. That's how a woman's body uses estrogen, and there is no superior model. By using E2 only, women are missing out on the benefits conferred by other estrogen compounds, particularly the potent health protections that E3 delivers.

The pharmaceutical companies and their supporters want you

to believe all hormone replacement is the same, that the risks associated with chemicalized estrogen are risks that extend to bioidentical estrogen as well. In my experience, this is simply not true.

A Reminder: Always Pair Estrogen with Progesterone

No estrogen—chemicalized or bioidentical—is safe to use on its own for long-term hormone replacement. The balance that progesterone provides to estrogen is critical. Without progesterone—or, unbalanced by progesterone—estrogen over time will increase the likelihood of developing uterine cancer. To be used safely, supplemental estrogen must be accompanied by progesterone.

The Benefits and Safety of Bioidentical Hormones

I believe that bioidentical hormones are safe and beneficial for women who are suffering from a loss of estrogen. I know this from the testimony and medical results of thousands of patients. As my patient Irene told me, "I feel so good now. I finally sleep at night. I no longer need three glasses of wine to destress. And my vagina feels like celebrating." Theresa, who'd been reluctant to commit to HRT treatment, said, after three months of taking it, "I know this is working. I feel so good, so healthy."

I can go on and on sharing success stories from my patients. Yes, my happy, healthy patients are proof of both the benefits and the safety of bioidentical HRT. The growing collection of peer-reviewed research studies also points to its efficacy and safety. In one large, significant study (called the E3N cohort study) of more than fifty thousand Frenchwomen, researchers compared different groups of women over an eight-year period: women who were not using any form of HRT, women who were using chemicalized progestin, and those who were using bioidentical progesterone. The group using the chemical HRT showed an increase in breast cancer, whereas those women who used bioidentical HRT had a 10 percent decrease in breast cancer. The researchers then tested the use of estrogen plus progesterone, in both chemical and bioidentical forms. The same relative results were found. The most startling finding, however, was that women who used no hormones at all experienced a sixfold higher incidence of breast cancer compared with the women who received bioidentical hormone treatment, emphasizing again that it's better to take some HRT than none at all.

The research is solid and ever growing: bioidentical estrogen and other bioidentical hormones have not been shown to increase risks for breast cancer—and researchers have actually seen evidence that they decrease risk for the disease. Bioidentical hormones can help to protect heart health, not jeopardize it.

Bioidentical hormones are my standard for "natural" hormone replacement therapy. I wish they were the pharmaceutical industry standard, too, but they are not. The big drug manufacturers do not appear to be set up to produce or profit from bioidentical hormones. Although there are a few brand-name bioidentical supplements on the market, such as Vivelle, Estrace, or Alora, I do not believe that these pharmaceutical products contain all types of estrogen a woman needs. Typically they contain estradiol but not estriol (used to balance the effect of estradiol). The patches that are offered don't meet the minimum amount of hormone for proper absorption; in other words, no one prescription product will deliver all the estrogen that you need.

Of course, you need to know your own hormonal profile and

learn how to help your health care provider determine your specific hormonal and supplement needs. I will cover that in chapter 6. The "right" dosage is always about what you require as an individual; a one-size-fits-all approach will rarely if ever meet your specific needs.

YOUR HEALTH JOURNAL

As you become more familiar with the factors underlying your hormonal health, it's crucial that you pay attention to yourself, to your moods and physical symptoms. I recommend keeping an almost daily record. This can be in a journal, a notes section on your smartphone, an audio recording—whatever works for you. Think of your journal as a place where you can record your thoughts and feelings, questions you might have, and any notes about yourself. I encourage all my patients to keep this kind of log so they can begin to cue in to their bodies and moods; patterns will begin to emerge over the course of a month or so. These records will become a vital source of information when you connect with a physician for treatment.

Take some time to reflect on where you are now by responding to the following questions.

- If you are still getting your period, is it regular or erratic?
- Do you notice an increased interest in sex at time of ovulation?
- Do you notice a lull right before you bleed?
- If you no longer get your period, when did it stop?
- Are you experiencing night sweats?
- Are you experiencing hot flashes during the day?

- Are you more irritable or anxious than usual, or have these feelings become your new normal?
- Has your sleep pattern changed? Is your sleep disrupted? If so, how?

Next, review signs of estrogen deficiency and excessive estrogen and note in your journal any that may apply to you.

Signs of Estrogen Deficiency

Mental fogginess

Forgetfulness

Difficulty staying focused

Depression

Anxiety

Mood swings

Difficulty falling asleep

Waking up in the middle of the night and inability to go back to sleep

Hot flashes

Night sweats

Temperature swings

Extreme fatigue

Reduced energy or stamina

Decreased interest in sex

Dry eyes

Dry skin

Dry vagina

Erratic monthly cycle

Sagging breasts

Pain with sex

Weight gain, especially around the middle

Increase in joint pain—knees and hips especially

Increase in headaches

Episodes of rapid heartbeat

Frequent bloating

Feeling invisible

Signs of Excess Estrogen

Breast tenderness or pain, especially around the nipple

Increase in breast size

Water retention (edema in fingers and ankles)

Pelvic cramps

Nausea

Cold hands and feet

Weight gain

Change to your monthly cycle (more frequent bleeding)

Keep in mind that these symptoms can have multiple causes, not all related to estrogen or other hormonal deficiency. However, as a general, easy rule to follow, start by understanding your own estrogen levels. If you are deficient, then you know these symptoms have a hormonal component.

2

Estrogen Is Not the Enemy

A year or so ago, a new patient came into my office, sat down across from me, and said, "Dr. Reiss, I feel so invisible."

Audrey's voice sounded sad and hopeless. Her face looked wan, drained of color and vigor. She seemed both agitated and depleted and looked uncomfortable in her body, as if just sitting there took effort. Strain lined her face. I could see that she was in pain, both physically and emotionally. I didn't have her chart in front of me, but as I looked at her, I guessed that she was somewhere in her midfifties.

It turns out Audrey was only forty-five. As we sat together, Audrey described how she'd been feeling for the past couple of years. She was carrying extra weight around her middle, shoulders, and arms—pounds that she couldn't shed, no matter what diet she tried. She felt anxious a great deal of the time, as if her emotions were "hijacked by some kind of impostor." She felt tired, sluggish, down in the dumps, and "deeply unsexy," she told me.

She'd almost resigned herself to the conclusion that this medley of symptoms was what aging was about. Almost. Part of her had not given up hope and somehow knew it just wasn't okay to feel as she was. Part of her knew she deserved better. So here she was, sitting in front of me, looking for answers, seeking solutions.

Have you ever felt invisible like my patient? Do you struggle with low moods or anxiety? Do you feel tired much of the time, like you no longer have energy to exercise, never mind start new projects or participate in your usual activities? Maybe you also feel a new kind of achiness in your bones and joints. Or that your life as a sensual, sexually attractive woman is over for good. Do you wonder if you'll ever get a full night's sleep again?

If so, you are not alone. **Millions of women like Audrey—and perhaps you—are suffering from the debilitating effects of estrogen deficiency, including foggy brain, low energy, low sex drive, and weight gain, and from other kinds of hormonal imbalance.** Women low in estrogen can be frustrated, scared, and ashamed of how they feel. The good news is that these negative, undermining feelings are often completely avoidable.

So let me ask you another question. Do you think hormone replacement therapy is good or bad for you?

If you think you've heard that it's "bad" for you and dangerous to your health, you are also not alone. Most women have heard only inaccurate, incomplete, and outdated information about HRT based on a flawed and misinterpreted study from 2002.

Behind the Fear: A Brief History of HRT

The fear that shadows HRT can be traced back to an exact moment in time: when the 2002 Women's Health Initiative study, or WHI, was first published. Originally, the WHI was planned as an eight-year study of the effects—good or bad—of HRT. But when study leaders began to see an increase in breast cancer among study participants, they not only suspended the study but also went public with these findings. Almost overnight, many women were told by their physicians to ditch their hormonal therapy. In a matter of weeks, millions of women flushed their medicines down the toilet—sometimes without even consulting their physicians.

Now, eighteen years since the WHI study, we know that, although the study's intentions were good, its design as well as the early inferences from it were seriously flawed; indeed, in my opinion, and as I will show soon, the study design was intentionally skewed and its principal investigators interpreted the data in line with a specific agenda. However, before we delve deeper into all that went wrong with the WHI study and its aftermath, let's take a moment to look at how menopause and perimenopause were treated in the years and decades *before* WHI to understand more of the background on hormones.

Hormone replacement therapy began to be prescribed to women in the United States in the 1930s to assuage symptoms of menopause. These early forms of hormones were by and large chemicalized estrogen. (Bioidentical estrogen, the safer and more effective option, also existed, but it was not easy to procure, and its system of delivery—by injection—made it difficult to administer and unappealing to many women.)

In these early decades, women using hormone replacement therapy were taking estrogen only, not the combination of synthetic estrogen and progesterone that would be developed later. Still, women enjoyed many of the benefits of estrogen therapy— they slept better, their skin retained its elasticity, and their hot flashes and night sweats disappeared or were reduced. They also received some of the disease-preventing benefits of supplemental estrogen, including significant protection against cardiovascular disease. Indeed, hormonal therapy was considered a best practice in the treatment of breast cancer, before drug therapies, such as tamoxifen, were even discovered.

In the 1960s and early 1970s, HRT use soared, but by the mid-1970s, side effects, including uterine cancer, began to be observed. These disturbing findings led to two major changes in hormone replacement therapy. First, many women stopped taking chemicalized estrogen to reduce their cancer risk. Second, HRT drugmakers began pairing chemicalized estrogen with a chemicalized progesterone in order to counteract the elevated cancer risk posed by estrogen used on its own. By the 1980s, the addition of chemicalized progesterone brought many women back to HRT, with some reverting to chemicalized hormone replacement therapy.

During these years, bioidentical estrogen and other bioidentical hormones were quietly but steadily gaining use, even though many in the medical community dismissed them as ineffective compared with big pharma's synthetic versions. But women were drawn to this natural alternative, especially when they discovered that they did not have to take an injection. Indeed, I began prescribing bioidentical hormones in 1982, not long after I started my medical practice, and have continued to this day.

The Great Flush

In 1998, when the WHI began collecting data on over sixteen thousand women from forty health centers around the United States, the participating women were taking one or two of the most commonly prescribed medications, such as Premarin, a chemicalized version of estrogen, and Provera, a chemicalized substitute for progesterone. Some women in the study received a regimen of hormone replacement therapy using Premarin and Provera. In a separate study track, women received only Premarin. Still others received a placebo. Investigators planned for the health-tracking phase of the study to be about eight years, but the WHI did not last that long.

Approximately five years into the study, researchers halted the study abruptly, because women who were using Premarin and Provera were showing signs of several health risks, including breast cancer, coronary heart disease, stroke, and pulmonary embolism. The researchers were surprised and concerned. Indeed, the WHI data were found to "convincingly support a direct association between decreasing hormone therapy use and declining breast cancer incidence." However, these supposed findings were not only taken out of context but also critically misinterpreted.

The most significant flaw in the WHI findings involved the study population. The more than 16,000 women who were enrolled in the study ranged in age between 50 and 79, with an average age being slightly over 63 years. In addition, 50 percent of these women were obese and smokers. This age range matters, because a great many of the women in the study weren't just menopausal— they were ten or even twenty years *beyond* initial menopause. Their bodies had been without sufficient estrogen for years, which itself raised their risks for breast cancer, cardiovascular disease, and other serious conditions. In other words, when older, postmenopausal women go more than ten years in low estrogen, they naturally become more vulnerable to developing breast cancer and cardiovascular disease.

The younger women in the WHI study, women in their fifties who had not been without estrogen for as long as the older women, *did not show the risks for breast cancer.* Indeed, since the time of the initial WHI results, other research has shown that women who began supplementing with estrogen and progesterone *within ten* years of menopause *had lower risks of cardiovascular disease* and overall mortality. Further, even the original WHI data showed clearly that the women who used only estrogen (Premarin) had a 23 percent *reduction* in breast cancer.

In the years since 2002, the WHI has been criticized for failing to calculate how women's risks of developing disease shift over time: the older women are and the longer they are postmenopausal, the higher their overall disease risk. Since then, two independent European researchers reexamined the original WHI data using different statistical measurements and again found that there was no increased risk of breast cancer with HRT use.

Unfortunately, the news media reported on the misleading results of the WHI in stories that emphasized the finding that there was a link between breast cancer and estrogen supplements. They scared everybody—patients, physicians, and other scientists—and led them to believe that estrogen was risky and dangerous. From that time to today, physicians have been discouraging women who are candidates for HRT from using estrogen and other hormones to help with menopausal and perimenopausal symptoms. Many physicians still take the erroneous position that *all* hormonal therapy is dangerous and carries significant risk of causing breast cancer, among other diseases.

However, perhaps the most egregious part of this whole story— the WHI study gone wrong—is that after its data was correctly interpreted, it was revealed that at the outset of the WHI, its choice of design was intentionally biased. The scientists chose older, overweight women, perhaps because they believed HRT was not good. Then, when the data was not to their liking, it appears that they skewed the interpretations and published erroneous results. In their book, *Estrogen Matters*, Avrum Bluming, M.D., and Carol Tavris, Ph.D., present damning evidence of unprofessional and unethical conduct. Indeed, they cite that in 2014, Dr. Samuel Shapiro and colleagues conducted an "in-depth analysis" of the WHI study, its results, and the conduct of the leading scientists. As Bluming and Tavris point out, Shapiro and his colleagues stated unequivocally, "the over-interpretation and misinterpretation of the findings in the

WHI study has resulted in major damage to the health and well-being of menopausal women. . . . [T]he claim that the 'findings do not support the use of this therapy for chronic disease prevention' is not defensible."

Bluming and Tavris go on further to scrutinize the conduct of some of the scientists, revealing that one of the "insiders," Dr. Robert Langer, admitted in 2017 that "highly unusual circumstances prevailed when the WHI trial was stopped prematurely in July 2002. The investigators most capable of correcting the critical misinterpretations of the data were actively excluded from the writing and dissemination activities."

Bluming and Tavris point out that the handling of the data and its release to the press in an inaccurate, misleading form "violated key scientific conventions: statistical accuracy, co-author review, and publication in a professional journal before the hoopla of press releases and other publicity." They then conclude that the principal investigators of WHI "had an agenda from the outset": to "show that [hormones] were harmful."

Sadly, one researcher has quantified the impact of this mass abandonment of estrogen, estimating that as many as ninety-eight thousand women may have died prematurely as a consequence of stopping or avoiding hormone replacement therapy. (This number was arrived at by counting a quarter of the women who stopped taking estrogen.) In the meantime, women have been deprived of the benefits and protections that estrogen, especially bioidentical, confers. And without any additional estrogen supplements, they are at greater risk for the very conditions—including breast cancer and heart disease—that they sought to protect themselves against by stopping estrogen therapy in the aftermath of the WHI study.

Yet the most important takeaway from the WHI is that estrogen actually has the power to *decrease* the risk of breast cancer.

But some of us already knew this. In 2001, a year before the WHI results were released, another report was published about hormone replacement therapy. It was exhaustive and painstakingly researched—and yet it received none of the fanfare or attention that the WHI results received later. Dr. Trudy Bush, a brilliant, highly respected, and nationally recognized epidemiologist and specialist in women's health, then a professor at the University of Maryland Medical School and an adjunct professor at Johns Hopkins University, conducted a deep and thorough analysis of twenty-five years of scientific research into the use of hormone replacement therapy, including a review of fifty studies on the subject over a twenty-five-year period. Her study looked at the various combinations of estrogen only and estrogen and progesterone. Dr. Bush concluded that *there was no evidence to link estrogen to breast cancer risk.*

Dr. Bush's rigorous and thorough study should have delivered a tremendous boost of confidence, encouragement, reassurance, and clarity for women and for the doctors helping guide their health care and hormone-treatment decisions. Instead, a year later, the widely publicized WHI study spread fear and confusion that persists today.

Isn't It Natural to Lose Estrogen?

I am asked this question almost every day. Let me start by asking you another question: Isn't it "natural" for some people to have less than perfect vision? Isn't it also perfectly acceptable, encouraged, and recommended that people with less than 20/20 vision wear glasses or contact lenses? I doubt any one of you would debate the effectiveness and desirability of "adjusting" your vision through eyeglasses or contact lenses.

The same goes for estrogen deficiency.

The belief that you ought simply to accept the decline of estrogen doesn't make sense. Just as wearing glasses improves your vision, supplementing with bioidentical hormones improves your overall well-being. Why should you be asked to "toughen up" and learn to live with symptoms that rob you of your spunk and vitality?

You shouldn't.

You can age with power and grace, sensuality and sexuality. And, even more important, you can boost your body's immunity, metabolism, and brain power.

Men are considered entitled to health and a high quality of life, and their ability to experience life fully is regarded as hugely important. Men are supported and encouraged to use testosterone supplements, as well as Viagra, by their doctors, their friends, and of course the companies selling these products. Women deserve no less support to feel well, to be sexually active and fulfilled.

This wake-up call about estrogen is long overdue. Too many women feel invisible. Too many women feel depleted and estranged from their essential selves. And the health of too many women is at risk because they do not know the good news about estrogen and other bioidentical hormones they can take to meet their individual needs.

In the pages ahead, I am going to cut through that confusion and fear and help you find the right hormone therapy for you. I will help you learn

- Effective ways to use hormonal therapy that will not only alleviate but eliminate hormonal disruptions such as PMS or the side effects of perimenopause or menopause
- How your particular levels of estrogen, progesterone, testosterone, and other hormones are affecting how you look and feel

- Which everyday habits—what you eat, drink, and wear—make you more likely to develop disease and ill health
- The risks and treatment options related to breast cancer.

I want to help you tune in to yourself and your own needs so that you can take charge and make informed decisions about your health. I feel it's my obligation as a women's doctor to break through the fear and misinformation so that you can make your own choices about how you want to live. Please consider that many women who don't yet have symptoms are slowly but surely developing underlying conditions that set them up for premature aging, illness, and even disease because of how their bodies are already responding to a gradual depletion of estrogen. I don't want you to be among these unsuspecting women who may be unaware that, each month, their bones can begin to weaken, their skin and vaginas can become more dry, their entire cardiovascular system may lose its protection from estrogen, and their brains can begin to lose vitality.

To further complicate matters, the impact of the decline in estrogen is now more severe because of the interplay of environmental and epigenetic stressors. Epigenetic refers to how our genes respond to our lifestyle and/or the environment in which we live. What do I mean? What you eat, the products you use, and the overall healthiness of your lifestyle have an enormous impact on both your hormonal health and your ability to fight or suppress disease. Yes, we all have genetic markers, strengths and vulnerabilities that we've inherited. However, depending on how we live, our genes can either be expressed . . . or not. For instance, you might inherit a vulnerability for a certain type of skin cancer. But you may not develop the disease if you take good care to protect your skin. This might seem like an oversimplification, and yet the basic truth remains: you have much more control over your health than you realize. For instance, a diet high in sugar and starch and a lack of regular exercise can damage the body and brain. Many chemicals used in cosmetics, household products, and even furniture act as endocrine disruptors, mimicking estrogen and "tricking" the body into thinking it has sufficient amounts of the hormone. The result? The body has a false sense that it has a lot of estrogen, so it begins to make less and less. These environmental disruptors are at the root of why even young women in their twenties are showing up in my office, feeling and acting as if they are in menopause.

It's time for you to get *the good news* about estrogen—so that you, and all the women you care about, can understand exactly how estrogen functions in your body and what benefits it can give you when supplemented in natural, bioidentical form. I also want to share the risks associated with using chemicalized estrogen and what steps you can take to reduce the harmful side effects, if you choose to use chemicalized estrogen.

As a twenty-first-century woman, you will live longer than previous generations. Indeed, it's been estimated that you will spend up to 40 percent of your life in menopause. I want you to know how you can protect your health and live a full, vital life without being hampered by the unnecessary effects of a loss of estrogen, which can be so easily remedied.

YOUR HEALTH JOURNAL: YOU'RE IN CHARGE

As you ready yourself to take charge of your health, it will be helpful to think about your goals, as well as where you are now. With that in mind, please answer some questions about where you are now:

1. Do you want to improve the way you feel? If so, how?
2. Would you like to improve the way you look? If so, how?
3. Are you currently dealing with one or more health situations?
4. Are you open to speaking to a physician or other health care practitioner about bioidentical hormonal treatment?

Keep in mind your responses to these questions. They will help you as you continue to familiarize yourself with your hormonal health and build sufficient background to make informed decisions about your health care with your physician or health care practitioner.

3

The Interplay of Hormones

Estrogen is the conductor of your body-brain symphony, but several other important hormones are supporting players, helping you stay in hormonal balance. In this chapter, I will summarize the main functions of these hormones and highlight how they interact with or support estrogen and help your overall hormonal health. As you will see, many of these hormones—from progesterone and thyroid hormones to testosterone to DHEA and melatonin—are integral to your feeling and looking your best. And when it comes to taking steps to begin a regimen of bioidentical hormone treatment, you will want to consider how these other hormones come into play. Indeed, many women can benefit from additional hormonal therapy treatment that targets the problems caused by deficiency or imbalance of these other hormones. Again, keep track of any symptoms that you may be feeling; record your notes in your journal so that your hormonal profile stays up to date and complete.

Knowing What to Look For

Stephanie first came to see me when she was fifteen. Her mother brought her in to the office because, since getting her period at twelve, she'd been bleeding irregularly every few months. Her mother's main concerns were Stephanie's steady weight gain and the continued increase in her breast size. Her irregular period meant that she was not ovulating regularly, so I knew that the bleeding was tied to a condition called unopposed estrogen, which occurs after a very prolonged exposure to estrogen without the presence of sufficient progesterone. When I examined her and analyzed her tests, I found that Stephanie was indeed low in progesterone. In order to trigger the brain to ovulate regularly, Stephanie began a brief course of 10 percent progesterone cream. This small amount worked to stimulate ovulation and synchronize her body's other hormonal cycles. After a year, she was able to stop using the progesterone cream, as her body had rebalanced itself.

Infrequently, however, progesterone levels can work in a paradoxical manner. Terry was one such case. She came to see me because she was experiencing increased anxiety, breast pain, water retention, and strange food cravings (pineapple! pickles! green peppers!). Curiously, these are all fairly common signs of low progesterone. Initially, I treated Terry in the same way as I did Stephanie. But given her age (thirty-six), I wanted to carefully monitor her estrogen and progesterone levels once she started using the progesterone cream, to make sure that her estrogen levels did not escalate. Unopposed estrogen in perimenopausal and menopausal women can trigger uterine cancer. At first, we were not sure of Terry's naturally occurring estrogen levels. Once she began the progesterone supplement, if she began to menstruate again regularly, then we'd know that her estrogen and progesterone were in balance. If she didn't menstruate, then we'd know she also needed estrogen supplementation. And finally, if she began to menstruate irregularly (like Stephanie), then we'd know that Terry had actually developed unopposed estrogen.

As I've mentioned, each of you is an individual and needs to be treated as such. As you gather information that goes into your hormonal profile and share these details with your physician or health care provider, you will want to keep in mind that it takes time to build a complete understanding of what supplements you need and what are the best combinations for your particular situation. Tracking your own symptoms can help you pay attention to the overlap of the signs of deficiency and/or excess of various hormones. Ultimately, you and your physician will be able to narrow down exactly what you need—and what you don't—in order to bring you into optimal hormonal balance.

Progesterone

Progesterone, second to estrogen in importance to women's health, is the perfect dance partner for estrogen. Progesterone helps balance the dominance of estrogen, in part by converting estradiol (E2) to estrone (E1), a significantly weaker estrogen compound. Early in a woman's life, progesterone supports fertility and enables conception. Estrogen and progesterone work in tandem to support reproduction. Progesterone is very low for the first two weeks of the cycle and then increases substantially after ovulation. Progesterone prepares the uterus for conception and to carry a pregnancy successfully by triggering the thickening of the uterine lining.

Throughout your life, progesterone supplies you with energy and focus while simultaneously encouraging feelings of calm, control, and ease. In addition, progesterone offers powerful protection against breast cancer by reducing estrogen receptors in the breast and by slowing the rate of breast cell growth. A landmark study at Johns Hopkins University showed that women with low progesterone had more than five times the risk of developing breast cancer during perimenopause than did women with normal progesterone levels, as well as significantly greater risk of dying from the disease. Other studies have shown that women with breast cancer who have surgery while their bodies are producing progesterone (during the two weeks following ovulation) have higher survival rates than women whose surgeries happen when their bodies aren't producing much progesterone.

Progesterone reduces and controls inflammation and protects against atherosclerosis, helps maintain healthy brain function, increases the production of myelin (a substance that shields and protects nerves in the brain and throughout the central nervous system), and helps prevent or allay depression and anxiety by stimulating production of GABA, a neurotransmitter that promotes calm and relaxation. GABA and progesterone also encourage sleep.

Here's a quick quiz to see if you might be experiencing progesterone deficiency:

- Do you have irregular periods?
- Have you stopped getting your period altogether, though you think you're too young to be in menopause?
- Do you spot before your period?
- Are your menstrual cramps worsening?
- Have your periods become heavier?
- Do you experience breast pain before your period begins?
- Have your breasts suddenly increased in size?
- Have you ever been diagnosed with endometriosis or fibroids?
- Have you experienced poor quality of sleep before or during your periods?
- Have you been prescribed birth control pills to "regulate" your period?

If you answered yes to any of the above, keep track and share this information with your doctor.

A Caveat About Progesterone

If you are already taking progesterone or considering it, you should be aware that it has potentially complex effects. About 10 percent of women can have a paradoxical response to progesterone. Most women experience a calming effect, and it promotes sleep, but a small percentage of women will get agitated. Most women experience a decrease in food cravings, but a minority of women complain of an increase in appetite and cravings. Further, while progesterone usually acts as a diuretic, it makes some women retain water. For women who have a lot of yeast (if, for example, you suffer from candida), progesterone can increase bloating. These side effects are considered mild from a medical point of view, but my patients who fall into this group find them annoying, to say the least. If you have any of these reactions, you need to have a yearly ultrasound to make sure the lining of the uterus does not become too thin or too thick—ideally it should measure under 5mm.

Uses for Bioidentical Progesterone

PMS
Postpartum depression
Irregular periods
Immunity boost
Hearing loss

Seizures

Allergies

Irritable bowel syndrome (IBS)

Interstitial cystitis

Endometriosis

Cycle-related fertility problems

Sleep problems

Water retention

Testosterone

Testosterone, popularly thought of as a male hormone, serves many important functions in a woman's body. Testosterone, mostly produced in the ovaries, peaks in production when you are in your early twenties and decreases by nearly 50 percent by the time you reach your midforties. In healthy amounts, testosterone supports sexual functioning, including arousal and response, and the ability to experience an orgasm and other forms of sensual pleasure. In your reproductive cycle, testosterone supports follicle development, an essential component of successful conception. This hormone also imbues women with feelings of confidence. Research has shown that it reduces the physiological reaction to fear (a wired-in threat response). You know those sweaty palms, rapid heart rate, and overall nervous feeling you get when encountering a frightening situation? Testosterone lessens the intensity of this response in women. Sufficient levels of testosterone help limit and quiet fear and timidity, providing an internal sense of safety, security, and strength.

Testosterone also helps build and strengthen muscles. It reduces muscle fatigue and boosts physical performance in ways that enhance athletic ability as well as balance and eye-hand coordination. It also supports and protects bone health, lifts mood, and alleviates depression. When you have sufficient levels of testosterone, you tend to have an overall sense of well-being, along with sexual desire and confidence. These feelings can often successfully allay depressive feelings. Finally, testosterone protects healthy blood vessels by helping produce nitric oxide, and it prevents plaque from forming in blood vessels, protecting you from developing the precursors to heart disease.

Many women are not aware that they might have a deficiency or excess of testosterone.

Respond to the following questions to see whether you have too much or too little.

- Have you lost a sense of excitement about your life?
- Do you feel more insecure in your dealing with work or relationships?
- Do you have difficulty setting boundaries and sticking up for yourself?
- Have you recently lost muscle mass or gained weight?
- Have you lost interest in being sexually active?
- Are your nipples and/or clitoris less sensitive than they used to be?
- Does it take longer for you to reach orgasm?
- Is your pubic hair thinning?

If you responded yes to more than three of these questions, then you might be in a low testosterone state and could benefit from bioidentical supplements. Please answer these questions:

- Is your facial skin oilier than usual?
- Do you have acne?

- Do you feel exceptionally agitated before and during your period?
- If you no longer get your period, do you feel more aggressive when in a surprising or threatening situation?
- Do you often feel on edge, as if you're on the defensive?

If you answered yes to one or more of these questions, you might have excessive testosterone. When you get your blood work done (see chapter 6 for further details), ask your physician or health care provider to ascertain your levels of testosterone as well as other hormones. If you find that you have excessive testosterone, you will need to understand more about what is causing it. Possible root causes include an imbalance between your estrogen and progesterone levels, insulin or leptin resistance, thyroid issues, and adrenal fatigue. As I have seen in my patients, high testosterone can be managed safely and naturally through both bio-identical supplementation and changes in your diet and exercise. (See chapter 7 for these suggestions.) However, keep in mind that testosterone cannot be measured in the blood, only at the cellular level. So certain test results can be deceiving; make sure testosterone is measured accurately.

Uses for Testosterone
- Treat infertility
- Promote bone growth and protect bone health
- Treat depression
- Restore sexual function and heighten sexual gratification and orgasm
- Treat prolapse of rectum and bladder, a common consequence of hysterectomy
- Alleviate stress incontinence

Testosterone Side Effects

- Aggressive, impatient behavior
- Acne on the face and/or body
- Receding hairline at the front and top of head and facial hair growth
- Hair growth only at the site of application, if using a bioidentical gel or cream

The side effects of bioidentical testosterone use are usually related to an excess of testosterone and can be remedied by adjusting the dose.

Myths About Testosterone

Many women are reluctant to use bioidentical testosterone, afraid that it will promote a masculine appearance. The truth is that when testosterone is used appropriately, it won't make you grow body hair, develop stocky, masculine muscles, or otherwise look like a man. Testosterone can, however, boost sexuality and sex drive, give you a sense of inner power and confidence, enhance feelings of worth and well-being, and make you physically stronger and more athletic. Other benefits can include an improvement in visual and spatial memory and a reduction of apolipoprotein, commonly called bad cholesterol and associated with the development of Alzheimer's.

Estrogen's Shepherd: SHBG

Estrogen exerts a significant influence over several other hormones by virtue of its relation to a protein called sex hormone–binding globulin, or SHBG. This protein helps regulate estrogen levels in the blood and is one of a fleet of similar proteins produced in the liver to help the body maintain hormonal balance. SHBG acts like estrogen's shepherd and minder, escorting estrogen through the bloodstream to cells and preventing estrogen levels from rising too high or falling too low. When estrogen levels climb too high, the liver generates more SHBG, which binds to estrogen and deactivates the hormone. When estrogen levels are low, the liver reduces production of SHBG, allowing more estrogen to move freely.

But SHBG doesn't bind only to estrogen—it also binds to and deactivates several other hormones, including thyroid hormone, human growth hormone, and testosterone. An excess of estrogen leads to an elevation of SHBG, which in turn leads to an increased binding up of these other hormones, leaving less of them available for the body to use. Low estrogen, on the other hand, frees up more of the other hormones affected by SHBG.

SHBG also interacts with testosterone. Indeed, most of the testosterone in your body is regulated by your levels of SHBG, which binds or frees testosterone based on the amount of estrogen you have in your bloodstream. Thus, estrogen and testosterone have a largely inverse relationship. When estrogen levels drop at different points in your monthly cycle, testosterone levels rise. When estrogen levels rise and the body generates more SHBG, testosterone levels go down. This seesaw relationship between the two hormones repeats itself throughout your monthly cycle and over the duration of your lifetime. It may contribute to the "roller coaster" feeling that you experience at certain points in your cycle and life. It's important for you and your physician to check whether your SHBG levels are either too high or too low. In addition, SHBG levels are also impacted by other substances and interactions. For example, testosterone decreases SHBG. Olive oil, coffee, alcohol, and sugar increase SHBG. Boron, magnesium, vitamin D, zinc, omega fatty acids, and cortisone decrease

SHBG. Drugs such as benzodiazepines, metformin, and Clomid can increase SHBG.

Signs of Elevated SHBG
Dry skin
Vaginal dryness
Weight gain
Cold hands or feet
Fatigue

These symptoms of elevated SHBG don't happen alone—they are always related to other hormone levels. High SHBG often happens along with either estrogen or thyroid deficiency, for example.

Signs of Low SHBG
High testosterone
Hypothyroidism
Insulin resistance
Obesity
Cushing's syndrome

Human Growth Hormone

The body's natural growth hormone, human growth hormone (HGH), drives the biological maturation process from childhood to adulthood and promotes cell growth, renewal, and repair throughout your life. Produced by the pituitary gland, HGH increases until it reaches a peak at mid-adolescence, around age sixteen, but continues to provide important benefits throughout adulthood.

HGH has powerful systemic benefits, enhancing nearly every aspect of a woman's physiological health. As its name suggests, HGH promotes growth—not uncontrolled growth, and not growth where it is unwarranted. HGH spurs growth and regeneration in the body where it is expressly needed, and only there. A significant agent against aging and cellular degeneration, HGH also contributes to mental function. Healthy HGH levels provide a sense of motivation and possibility, which is also a powerful anti-aging force. HGH interacts with the neurotransmitter serotonin and increases your motivation to be proactive.

HGH also helps maintain muscle tone and influences the look, feel, and health of the skin. It is a powerful fat burner—particularly for fat that collects around the midsection. HGH increases levels of adiponectin, a protein hormone that is involved in metabolic processes, including glucose regulation and fatty acid oxidation. HGH works in conjunction with adiponectin to break down fat in the body.

For several decades, there has been a great deal of controversy about whether HGH supplementation contributes to cancer. I believe these concerns are unfounded. Studies show no increase in cancer rates among people who have been treated with HGH to correct a deficiency. For example, there is no evidence that children who are given HGH to promote growth develop cancer. Bioidentical HGH can strengthen the immune system and its cancer-fighting capabilities. Used properly, HGH does not trigger cancer; it helps the body ward it off. (People with cancer, however, should not take HGH, as it may exacerbate cancer-cell growth.) There also have been concerns that HGH contributes to increased risk for diabetes, but, again, in my experience, the opposite is true. Low-dose HGH helps the body use insulin more effectively; lowers blood sugar, cholesterol, and triglycerides; and promotes weight loss. The FDA has deemed HGH supplements safe for use in other contexts at much higher doses than I recommend (see chapter 7 for a recommended range for supplement dosages). So if you are considering adding HGH to your regimen, consult with a physician who is experienced with hormone therapy and make sure to get regular follow-ups to confirm that your individual dosage is optimal and your levels of HGH are not interfering with other hormones' functions.

That said, some people should not take HGH, including cancer patients undergoing active treatment and people with adrenal exhaustion.

Take a look at the list below to see if you might be experiencing signs of HGH deficiency.

- Fatigue
- Anxiety, irritability
- Slow wound healing
- Difficulty sleeping
- Increased susceptibility to colds and flu
- Weight gain, especially around the core (waist and abdomen)
- Sagging skin on face and body
- Increased wrinkles
- Diminished enthusiasm and interest in new projects, ideas, and opportunities
- Lack of confidence
- Increased negativity
- Greater need for approval and reassurance from others

Again, many of these symptoms correspond to imbalances in other hormones, so ask your health care practitioner to measure your HGH levels to see if you might benefit from supplements.

DHEA

Dehydroepiandrosterone (DHEA) is the most abundant hormone in the body. DHEA can function, directly or indirectly, to protect against disease; boost energy, endurance, and mood; and slow the process—and the outward signs—of aging. The human body makes greater quantities of DHEA than it does any other hormone. Often regarded as a male hormone, DHEA is produced by women in abundance—and it is of vital importance to your overall health. DHEA functions like a master hormone in the body and is able to convert itself into other hormones—including estrogen—on an as-needed basis. It also boosts levels of several other hormones, including HGH and progesterone, and reduces levels of cortisol, the stress- and inflammation-triggering hormone.

DHEA has the capacity to increase levels of important proteins, such as PI3-kinase/Akt, which regulates glucose in the brain, protecting the brain from damage from excess glucose. DHEA is also a powerful natural antidepressant. I recommend it to my patients as a wellness hormone to lower stress. Indeed, it also acts as a powerful adaptogen—an agent that naturally helps the body protect itself from external or internal stress. (For more on adaptogens, see chapter 7.) DHEA protects against breast and other cancers, guards against cardiovascular disease, and improves overall immune functioning.

The influence of DHEA over health and wellness is so broad that to list its benefits would require a trip to every corner of the body. This adaptive hormone does the following:

- Promotes healthy thyroid function
- Maintains adrenal health
- Increases insulin sensitivity and lowers risk for diabetes
- Aids in weight loss, boosting levels of the fat-burning hormone adiponectin
- Eases depression, lowers anxiety, and promotes feelings of well-being
- Protects brain function, especially memory
- Enhances bone mass and muscle development

Recently, however, researchers and physicians like myself began observing that more and more women—and men—are producing less and less DHEA. The reasons are unclear, but the phenomenon is probably attributable to environmental influences, depletion of important vitamins and minerals in the soil and therefore our foods. So any chance you get, enjoy cruciferous vegetables, which are loaded with DHEA, and consider taking a supplement, which can also act as an adaptogen. (For more on supplements and other ways to improve your hormonal balance through nutrition, see chapter 7.)

Signs of DHEA Deficiency
Dry eyes, skin, and hair
Vaginal dryness
Extreme fatigue
Depression or mood swings
Problems with memory or focus
Noticeable decrease in sex drive
Loss of pubic hair

Pregnenolone

Pregnenolone was first identified in the 1950s as a treatment for rheumatoid arthritis because it acts like a naturally occurring steroid within the body. Soon after, however, cortisol (the stress hormone produced by the adrenal glands) was discovered to be a much more effective tool in treating arthritis, and thus pregnenolone was dropped as a treatment. Despite that early history, pregnenolone has recently been found by scientists to have many health benefits—both physically and mentally.

Our bodies naturally make pregnenolone through cholesterol, but as we age we begin to produce less and less of it. However, taken properly, it's an easy and safe supplement (made from wild yams) that can help increase mental focus, memory, and overall brainpower. My patients who take pregnenolone also notice an increase in their intellectual and social skills, alertness, and well-being. This powerful hormone also encourages new cell growth.

Pregnenolone also

- Eases joint pain and arthritis
- Lowers cholesterol
- Protects the eye's retina, improving perception of color and detail
- Supports fertility and pregnancy
- Raises alertness and confidence

Answer the following questions to see if you might benefit from optimizing your pregnenolone levels.

- Are you more forgetful lately?
- Have you experienced a loss of energy?
- Do you feel less motivated at work?
- Do you feel less able to concentrate?
- Is there a history of dementia or Alzheimer's disease in your family?
- Do you take anti-anxiety medication?
- Do you have difficulty seeing the vividness of colors?
- Do you have arthritis or joint pain?

Again, many of these questions overlap with those you are using to determine if you may have other hormonal imbalances; my point is to make sure that you are familiar with how pregnenolone functions and what can happen when it's low. Ask your physician to test for it so that you can determine whether you are deficient. Pregnenolone has been tested and used by many of my patients for years.

Thyroid Hormone

The thyroid is a small butterfly-shaped gland at the base of the throat, which you can feel just above the collarbone. The thyroid plays a central role in regulating the body's metabolism, setting and adjusting the metabolic rate of cells throughout the body. The thyroid gland uses iodine absorbed by the body to make two thyroid hormones: thyroxine (T4) and triiodothyronine (T3).

T4 is produced in higher quantities, while T3 is significantly more potent. The pituitary gland controls the thyroid and its hormone production by producing TSH (thyroid-stimulating hormone) in response to low T3 and T4 levels.

Thyroid problems are common in women, far more so than in men. Irregular thyroid function, with an excess or deficiency of thyroid hormones, causes significant, often debilitating, health problems for women, including weight and metabolic issues, extreme fatigue and difficulty sleeping, and depression and anxiety. Women between the ages of thirty and fifty are most likely to develop thyroid disorders, but they can occur in women both younger and older as well. Thankfully, more doctors are becoming aware of the need for thorough testing of thyroid hormones in the body. In the past, many thyroid issues went undetected and undiagnosed because of inaccurate and incomplete testing. To be sure that you receive a full screening, ask your physician for all three of the thyroid tests (see chapter 6 for test descriptions).

Several common thyroid conditions are autoimmune in nature, caused by abnormal behavior by the body's immune system. Immune cells attack healthy thyroid cells, impairing normal functioning of the gland and causing hormone levels to go awry. Graves' disease and Hashimoto's disease are two of the most common autoimmune thyroid disorders. Other causes include genetic predisposition, lack of iodine, and excessive exposure to pollutants and chemicals.

Thyroid disorders come in two general forms: hypothyroidism (low levels of one or more thyroid hormones) or hyperthyroidism (high levels of one or more thyroid hormones). Hypothyroidism is associated with increased risk for breast cancer and is often accompanied by depression. In fact, frequently the depression is identified before the thyroid imbalance. Women with hypothyroidism who are treated with antidepressants will most often not respond to these medications.

As you continue to create your own hormonal profile, it's important to obtain the tests for all the thyroid hormone levels. Take a look at the lists of symptoms below to see if you have any that might indicate either a high or low thyroid hormone.

Symptoms of Low Thyroid Hormone (Hypothyroidism)
- Low energy
- Fatigue—wake up slowly and in a bad mood
- Take long to sweat
- Poor hair and nails
- Weight gain, extreme difficulty losing weight
- Cognitive impairment, especially difficulty with memory
- Sensitivity to cold temperatures
- Swelling or bloating of the face and neck
- Widespread muscle and joint pain and stiffness
- Dry, flaky skin
- Constipation
- Decreased heart rate
- Frequent, irregular, and/or heavy periods
- Depression
- Cold hands and feet

Symptoms of Excess Thyroid Hormone (Hyperthyroidism)

- Weight loss that can be swift and unrelated to appetite and food consumption, which are likely to increase
- Fast heartbeat, irregular heartbeat, heart palpitations
- Trembling, especially apparent in fingers and hands
- Frequent, excessive sweating
- Sensitivity to warm temperatures
- Insomnia
- Anxiety
- Irritability, short-temperedness, aggression

Melatonin

Regarded primarily as a sleep-promoting hormone, melatonin has only recently begun to gain attention from physicians and scientists—most likely because so many of us battle sleep issues. What is clear, however, is that babies do not begin to produce melatonin until after age three months which is why infants don't sleep well at night and can benefit from breast-feeding to absorb the mother's melatonin and other vitamins. Once young children adapt to a circadian rhythm, melatonin production begins (controlled by the pineal gland). If you're a parent or grandparent, you will no doubt recall those first three to four months of babies *not* sleeping through the night!

Children ages one to three show the highest levels of melatonin. As we age, levels drop progressively by 80 percent. In senescent adults, these levels show an additional drop of some 10 percent. Scientists explain that the large drop in melatonin is probably the result of the increase in size of the human body, as well as the general interruption of our circadian rhythm due to the way we live now—not rising with the sun and not going to bed at sundown. However, the additional decline of melatonin as we age has not yet been fully explained.

The good news is that many people, including many of my own patients, have enjoyed significant health benefits with melatonin supplementation. Along with phototherapy (regulation of exposure to light and dark), melatonin works well to help people fall asleep and stay asleep. In particular, people who do shift work, who travel and suffer from jet lag, and who have other interruptions in their natural circadian rhythm have been helped by melatonin.

In addition to promoting restful sleep and helping regulate sleep-wake cycles, melatonin promotes cardiovascular health, guards the healthy function of the liver and kidneys, helps avoid bone loss, and delays and reverses alterations to levels of other hormones. Melatonin has also been shown to reduce inflammation and cut free radical load, promote metabolic health, and reduce cancer risk. It also works powerfully as an antioxidant in the brain, where it may slow or prevent the onset of Alzheimer's disease, since it limits beta-amyloid production, a protein dangerous to brain health and a marker for Alzheimer's disease.

Take a look at these signs of deficiency and excess to see if they apply to you:

Symptoms of Melatonin Deficiency
Poor sleep
Insomnia, waking during the night
Anxiety

Symptoms of Melatonin Excess
Sleepiness, grogginess
Nighttime alertness
Nightmares

As you think about your own physical and mental symptoms, don't feel that you need to be "tough" and endure the anxiety, depression, or loss of attention and focus that come with estrogen and other hormone deficiencies or excesses. If your physician seems resistant to discuss all that you can do to address your symptoms, seek a second opinion, preferably from a physician who is open to recommending bioidentical hormone replacement and better nutrition to alleviate your symptoms.

YOUR HEALTH JOURNAL: KEEPING IT ALL STRAIGHT

Take some time to review the chapter and its descriptions of hormones other than estrogen and potential imbalances that may apply to you. Make a list in your journal of any symptoms that you have noticed. This list will provide your health care practitioner with good information about your current health.

Part Two

. . . .

Estrogen Fallout

4

When Estrogen Declines: The Cascade Effect

When estrogen declines for any reason, including the gradual slowing of estrogen production that occurs with aging, a woman is at risk of developing a broad array of health issues. Understanding how estrogen keeps you healthy and vital is one of the first steps to owning your health. Let's take a look at what happens as estrogen begins to decline or becomes deficient and why considering bioidentical hormonal therapy can address and ameliorate symptoms, reverse certain conditions, and even protect against the development of certain diseases.

Estrogen Deficiency and Cardiovascular Disease

For all the years your body produces estrogen in relative abundance, your cardiovascular system benefits from significant protection against the precursors to heart disease, including hypertension, high blood pressure, and blood sugar imbalance. As estrogen declines, your risk for cardiovascular disease begins to climb. Heart disease claims the lives of more than 290,000 women in the United States each year. By the time you enter menopause, the estrogen buffer begins to disappear. Eventually, women's risks for heart attack and other forms of cardiovascular disease become roughly the same as those for men.

The loss of estrogen results in

- Increase in arterial sclerosis
- A 60 percent increase in aortal calcification
- Elevation of LDL, the "bad cholesterol"
- Increase of fibrinogen, which encourages the formation of blood clots
- Rise in blood pressure
- Decrease in vascular tone
- Significant increase in the incidence of heart attack and stroke

Taking bioidentical estrogen, along with progesterone, can protect you from developing cardiovascular disease by controlling blood pressure, preventing plaque from forming in arteries, managing levels of unhealthy cholesterol, and preventing the thickening of the heart wall. Estradiol, or E2, has particular importance to cardiovascular function and health. An abundant body of research has demonstrated that E2

- Helps regulate blood pressure
- Reduces levels of LDL
- Guards against heart failure
- Prevents plaque from forming in arteries
- Helps keep coronary arteries open by increasing the body's levels of nitrous oxide
- Lowers homocysteine, a marker for inflammation
- Reduces fibrinogen

Maintaining healthy levels of estrogen can contribute significantly to your cardiovascular function, as well as offer you protection against heart attack and stroke.

Estrogen's Role in Metabolism and Weight Management

One of the major reasons for weight gain in women throughout their forties and fifties (and even earlier) is dwindling estrogen levels. Too little estrogen can make you struggle to lose weight, even when you are making all the right choices in your diet and exercise. This weight struggle can be mentally and emotionally debilitating, as well as physically unhealthful. Indeed, many women think that estrogen replacement can cause weight gain—again, this is another misconception about HRT!

- Estrogen—especially estradiol (E2), the most powerful of the three estrogen compounds—exerts a powerful influence over metabolic health and is critical to weight management. Keeping estrogen levels healthy can help control appetite and prevent weight gain.
- Estrogen helps maintain levels of adiponectin, a protein that helps women shed fat. Adiponectin also helps regulate glucose levels, which is critical to maintaining metabolic health and function.
- Estrogen lowers levels of ghrelin, a hormone responsible for stimulating hunger and inducing food cravings, which can be intense and come about suddenly.
- Estrogen helps prevent binge eating because it functions as an appetite suppressant and plays an important role in regulating the brain's metabolism of energy. Estrogen also helps leptin—which promotes feelings of satiety—to work more effectively. Together, estrogen and leptin reduce food intake and provide a sense of fullness that curbs appetite.

Inflammation and How It Disrupts Your Body

Inflammation is a source of aging, a catalyst for disease, and a trigger for pain and discomfort throughout the body. That's not to say that inflammation is inherently bad or dangerous. The inflammatory response evolved for good reason. Inflammation serves an important function, mobilizing the immune system to respond to injury and the presence of foreign, potentially harmful substances. It's when inflammation becomes chronic and excessive that it causes problems, which can affect and undermine nearly every physiological system, organ, tissue, and cell in the body. From cancer and cardiovascular disease to osteoporosis and obesity, excess inflammation is a cause of and contributor to disease and dysfunction.

With people living longer than ever before, the long-term dangers of inflammation have become increasingly relevant to our health. Inflammation is the result of a mobilization of the immune system to neutralize a threat to the body, whether in the form of a virus or other pathogen, a chemical toxin or other environmental irritant, or an injury or trauma. Sometimes inflammation is perceptible—we can feel its effects in our stiff muscles and joints, our aching knees. Common symptoms of inflammation include the following:

- Pain and stiffness in joints, which may be worse in the morning
- Swelling, redness, feelings of warmth at joints
- Loss of mobility and flexibility
- Muscle stiffness
- Fatigue and lack of energy
- Fever and/or chills
- Nausea and vomiting

But inflammation often exists in the body without symptoms and without our awareness. This silent presence of inflammation is no less dangerous—in fact, it is more so. What causes inflammation? A lack of estrogen and other hormones is one significant factor, but there are other triggers of inflammation, including

- A diet high in sugar and starchy carbs
- Environmental exposure to toxins and chemicals
- Physical trauma and injury
- Chronic stress
- Poor sleep
- Viruses, bacteria, and germs that cause infection

It is impossible for any of us to shield ourselves completely from these inflammatory triggers, but you can do a lot to reduce excessive, chronic, and unhealthy inflammation by eating well, getting high-quality sleep, managing stress, and taking steps to minimize your exposure to chemical toxins. Bioidentical estrogen and other hormones can also help you limit inflammation and oxidative stress. Estrogen works as a powerful anti-inflammatory agent, increasing production of biochemicals that limit and reduce inflammation. One of estrogen's important tasks in a woman's body is its function as an antioxidant, limiting the proliferation of free radicals, which, along with making the body more vulnerable to cancer, further add to oxidative stress, exacerbating aging.

Free radicals create by-products, or oxidative stress, which, like inflammation, corrode the body and cause aging and disease. When a woman loses estrogen over the course of perimenopause and menopause, she loses a great deal of this protective antioxidant power. Without sufficient estrogen, women are more likely to experience excessive, aging, damaging inflammation—as well as the pain that often accompanies it. The pain and stiffness that many women experience during perimenopause and menopause is related to their declining hormones, including declines in estrogen.

Your Immune Response

Estrogen plays a significant role in the health, vitality, and function of your immune system, priming it to ward off infection and disease. As estrogen fluctuates and declines—whether during your monthly cycle, during and after pregnancy, or as part of perimenopause and menopause—your immune system can become vulnerable. Specifically, estrogen deficiency reduces levels of B cells and T cells, the workhorse cells of the immune system. Estrogen deficiency also increases levels of pro-inflammatory cytokines, which interfere with healthy immune function.

Women are disproportionately affected by autoimmune diseases. To date, researchers have identified more than 80 autoimmune diseases, and more than three-quarters of these diseases, such as multiple sclerosis, rheumatoid arthritis, Crohn's disease, and thyroid disorders, occur more often in women than in men. Over the past few decades, there has been a dramatic rise in autoimmune diseases—a disturbing trend that scientists cannot fully explain, and one that will continue to affect women in far greater numbers than men.

Besides declining estrogen and hormonal levels, other risk factors for disrupted immune function and autoimmune disease include genetics, lifestyle, and behavior (including stress, sleep, diet, and exercise, all of which are themselves affected by estrogen). Exposure to environmental toxins is also a likely culprit in the development of autoimmune disease. A woman's risk for autoimmune disease also increases as she ages, as does the risk of cancer, cardiovascular disease, and other diseases, in part because women are living longer than in previous generations.

All autoimmune diseases have one unifying characteristic: they are the result of the immune system turning on the body, attacking healthy cells rather than foreign invaders that pose a threat. While autoimmune diseases display a range of symptoms, several symptoms are common to many of them:

- Fatigue, often extreme and sometimes disabling
- Pain and stiffness, especially in joints
- Skin rashes
- Listlessness, a deep, persistent sense of being unwell, which can be disruptive to normal functioning

Estrogen protects your immune system. Women with chronically low estrogen and women who enter perimenopause or menopause earlier in life are at greater risk for developing some autoimmune diseases than are women who begin menopause later in life. If you already suffer from one or more immune disorders, continued low estrogen might worsen your situation. Multiple sclerosis, rheumatoid arthritis, and Sjögren's syndrome (which causes dry eyes and dry mouth) are some common autoimmune diseases exacerbated during menopause because of deficient estrogen.

Pregnancy, on the other hand, with its flood of estrogen, progesterone, and other hormones, frequently has a beneficial effect on autoimmune disease. Many women with autoimmune diseases such as multiple sclerosis and rheumatoid arthritis experience an alleviation or cessation of symptoms while they are pregnant and see a return or increase of symptoms after giving birth, which corresponds to falling levels of estrogen.

Estrogen stimulates the production of anti-inflammatory, immune-boosting cytokines, which in turn protect against and help alleviate and slow progression of certain autoimmune diseases. My patients who have multiple sclerosis, rheumatoid arthritis, Sjögren's syndrome, and other autoimmune diseases respond to estrogen treatment. If you are dealing with any one of these conditions, discuss with your physician how you can be helped with an HRT plan.

Memory, Cognitive Function, and Neurodegenerative Disease

Vivienne became my patient when she had turned sixty-five. A professor of art history at a nearby university, Vivienne had short white hair and piercing blue eyes. She had lived an interesting life—lecturing in Europe, the Middle East, and the United States on her specialty, Islamic art—and was well known for being a mesmerizing teacher.

Vivienne sought me out because she'd heard that I might be able to address her "slipping memory," as she described it. I would treat Vivienne for the last twenty years of her life. However, what we didn't know when Vivienne first came to see me was that she'd been in early menopause since she was in her late forties, when she began to have memory lapses, which now were worsening. Although she was able to stem the tide of total cognitive decline for the twenty years she was my patient, we were not able to eradicate all the damage already done. I can say with confidence that, had I met Vivienne when she first noticed her symptoms, she would have lived to see ninety with all her mental faculties intact.

Estrogen is essential to the overall health and function of your brain. Estrogen fuels and regulates brain activity, and it helps maintain the brain's structural health and integrity. Estrogen participates directly in supporting cognitive functions, protecting and enhancing learning and memory, alertness and focus, decision-making and planning. Estrogen is a major player in the dynamic biochemical balance of hormones, neurotransmitters, and other neurochemicals that affect every aspect of how a woman thinks, feels, and functions. Estrogen receptors throughout the brain's complex networks work with those neurotransmitters and other neurochemicals to process and stabilize memory, learning, and emotion.

Changes to estrogen levels affect mental clarity, the sharpness and responsiveness of mental function, and memory—often particularly verbal memory and spatial memory. Brief, temporary cognitive and mental deficits can be associated with low estrogen points in the monthly cycle. Feelings of mental fogginess or sluggishness, difficulty with word retrieval, and other symptoms of cognitive fatigue may occur when estrogen levels fall during the month. The overall gradual decline of estrogen during perimenopause and menopause often brings significant and lasting changes to the cognitive function and memory of women in middle age and beyond. Diminishing estrogen also increases the risk of developing neurodegenerative disease.

Estrogen exerts powerful effects over memory, learning processes, and other cognitive functions. Estrogen elevates production of several neurotransmitters (serotonin, norepinephrine, and dopamine, the chemical messengers that communicate between cells in the brain). These neurotransmitters influence memory and emotional processing. Estrogen supports brain plasticity and the formation of dendrites, tiny neural fibers that facilitate the brain's ability to process information.

Verbal facility and memory may change noticeably during menopause, when estrogen declines. Many women experience this symptom of menopause, the fumbling to remember a commonplace word, forgetting a person's name or the name of a street you drive along routinely. Almost every day, a new patient arrives telling me of her frustration at her cognitive decline.

Estrogen provides a crucial protection against deterioration of brain cells and loss of cognitive skills and memory. Estrogen increases BDNF, brain-derived neurotrophic factor, a neurochemical that helps brain cells survive longer and is essential to overall brain health. Estrogen also provides specific, powerful protection against the development of neurodegenerative disease, including Alzheimer's disease and Parkinson's disease, two of the most common neurodegenerative diseases for women. Indeed, women are twice as likely as men to develop Alzheimer's disease.

There is much we do not yet know about the catalysts for and development of neurodegenerative disease or about the factors that protect against it or make it worse. That said, there is tremendous evidence indicating that, for women, estrogen plays a significant role in protecting against or delaying neurodegeneration and the development of Alzheimer's and Parkinson's. Estrogen promotes healthy neural growth and repair and encourages and supports the growth of new brain cells. Estrogen also supports healthy blood flow to the brain and reduces beta-amyloid, a neurotoxic protein linked to Alzheimer's disease. Estrogen's stimulation of dopamine production and support for dopamine's effectiveness may guard against Parkinson's.

The anti-inflammatory powers of estrogen may be another form of protection against these neurodegenerative diseases—and the loss of this protection against inflammation when estrogen diminishes may be one way that estrogen influences women's risk of developing neurodegenerative disease. Women who use estrogen replacement therapy have significantly lower incidence of Alzheimer's disease.

Estrogen can not only prevent and slow the progression of neurodegenerative diseases but can also be used to treat them. The timing of estrogen therapy appears to make a significant difference in its ability to protect the brain and cognitive functions. Research suggests that estrogen therapy used during midlife, near the time of the initial, dramatic declines in estrogen during perimenopause and the beginning of menopause, has the greatest impact on long-term cognitive health. Estrogen therapy used later in life, after prolonged estrogen deficiency, may not be as effective in protecting and restoring cognitive function. In other words, memory loss that comes with estrogen deficiency may not be entirely recoverable, even after estrogen therapy is started.

Research also indicates that it isn't your age but the length of estrogen deficiency that affects the ability of supplemental estrogen to protect the hippocampus, a brain area critical to learning, memory, and emotion. (The earliest degeneration associated with Alzheimer's disease begins in the hippocampus.) The timing of estrogen therapy may also play a role in a woman's risk for Alzheimer's disease. While many studies show the protective effects of estrogen in reducing risk for Alzheimer's, there is also evidence that estrogen therapy has its most powerful protective effects against Alzheimer's when it is used early, at the beginning of menopause. Evidence also suggests that intermittent dosing of chemicalized estrogen may interfere with healthy cognition.

Bioidentical estrogen and other bioidentical hormones fortify and improve cognition, memory, and the structural health of the brain, without many of the risks posed by chemicalized hormone substitutes. As previously stated, they also can serve a critical purpose in slowing or preventing neurodegenerative diseases like Alzheimer's and Parkinson's.

- Estrogen protects brain tissue and the structural health of the brain.
- Estrogen increases blood flow to the brain.

- Estrogen protects and supports overall brain function, including the creation of new brain cells.
- Estrogen supports production of several neurotransmitters (such as serotonin, norepinephrine, acetylcholine, and dopamine) that influence thought and emotion.
- Estrogen (together with progesterone) improves cognitive control and attention in postmenopausal women.
- Estrogen protects against Alzheimer's disease and Parkinson's disease.

How Estrogen Affects Your Mood

Estrogen plays a significant role in regulating mood, preventing mood swings, and triggering or exacerbating depression and anxiety. When estrogen is low, you are likely to feel unmoored emotionally. You may feel you can no longer control, manage, or predict your emotions from one day, or even one hour, to the next. During the years before and throughout perimenopause and in early menopause, many of my patients complain of severe and erratic mood swings. They also experience an increase in a general, almost constant anxiety. Some women experience a creeping kind of depression that seeps into and sometimes dominates their lives. Not all women experience these, but anxiety, depression, and other mood problems become increasingly common with age—and the decline of estrogen contributes to that escalating risk.

Estrogen is critical to regulating mood. Specifically, estradiol (E2) is the estrogen compound that contributes most directly and effectively to regulating and balancing mood. The dips in mood that many women experience at points during their monthly cycles—days of feeling low, depleted, sometimes overcome with sadness—are largely due to natural drops in estrogen.

One of estrogen's important functions is as a monoamine oxidase (MAO) inhibitor. MAO is an enzyme that inactivates serotonin. By capping levels of MAO, estrogen enables serotonin and other mood-regulating neurotransmitters to remain active at healthy levels. Estrogen also works to control anxiety and panic attacks.

Depression

Estrogen is a powerful natural bulwark against depression. Insufficient estrogen can trigger depression even in women who might not otherwise be vulnerable to this debilitating emotional disorder. As mentioned, depression is more common for women in perimenopause and menopause, in large part because there is a diminishing supply of estrogen to balance and regulate mood. Fluctuating estrogen levels also affect mood and depression that are connected to pregnancy and childbirth. The plummeting of estrogen that occurs in the immediate aftermath of giving birth is one key factor that contributes to postpartum depression and, less frequently, to postpartum psychosis.

Major depression disorder (MDD) affects tens of millions of adults in the United States, causing hidden pain—and women suffer in greater numbers than men do. According to the National Institutes of Health, MDD afflicts slightly more than 8 percent of women in a given year, compared with 5 percent of men. Millions more women struggle with chronic or recurrent depressive symptoms that degrade their quality of life, interfere with their relationships, undercut their professional abilities, and diminish their energy and joy.

Bioidentical estrogen and other hormones are highly effective at alleviating depression in women—in my experience, far more so than conventional antidepressant pharmaceuticals. This is not to dismiss or discount the efficacy of these medications and their importance for many women who struggle with depression. However, while recognizing that SSRIs and other antidepressant drugs are necessary and sometimes lifesaving medications for women, I also believe they are overprescribed and overused, and their side effects not well understood. (See chapter 6 for more information on the impact of medications, including antibiotics.)

If you suffer from depression, taking bioidentical estrogen may provide significant protection and relief without some of the risks associated with conventional pharmaceutical depression treatment. While estrogen therapy for depression and other mood disorders won't be right for every woman, I believe it can be effective for many who are currently not being treated at all or who are being treated with medicines.

A word of caution: never go off medication or switch medications on your own without the close guidance and support of your physician.

Anxiety

Estrogen exerts significant influence over anxiety levels. Estrogen-related anxiety occurs as part of the monthly cycle, as well as during perimenopause and menopause. Postpartum anxiety is also related to the steep drop in estrogen after birth. Estrogen helps increase calming neurotransmitters, including serotonin and GABA, while regulating levels of norepinephrine and adrenaline, which have an excitatory effect. In this way, you can think of estrogen as having a balancing effect on your mood.

In the extreme, low estrogen can lead to panic attacks—a frightening form of anxiety that can lead to a disorder requiring a physician's care. The hallmark symptoms of panic attacks include a racing and/or irregular heartbeat, shortness of breath, chest pain, and intense feelings and sensations of fear and even terror. Although not common, some women in perimenopause experience panic attacks for the first time in their lives—though often these do not lead to a full-blown disorder. (Again, by understanding your body and how it changes over time and even within a particular month, you can cue in to these symptoms of anxiety and take steps to curtail the reactions so they don't develop into a more serious disorder.)

Specifically, estrogen helps regulate and stimulate production of several neurotransmitters that have positive, stabilizing effects on mood. Estrogen also stimulates production of serotonin, norepinephrine, dopamine, and GABA, important mood-regulating neurotransmitters.

Sleep's Effects on Mood, Depression, Anxiety, and Stress

If you are in perimenopause or in menopause, then you, like many of my patients, are probably experiencing difficulty sleeping; indeed, it's a hallmark of estrogen deficiency. Estrogen-related sleep problems are also common for women at points in their monthly cycle when estrogen is low. Regardless of her age or stage in life, when a woman has naturally low levels of estrogen or uses the low-dose chemicalized estrogen found in oral contraceptives, she is more likely to experience sleep difficulties.

Even women who have slept soundly and well for most of their lives can find themselves struggling to fall asleep and stay asleep as their estrogen levels fluctuate throughout perimenopause and menopause. Other symptoms of menopause, particularly night sweats, can intrude on sleep and be disruptive to sound nightly rest.

Sleep problems and mood problems go hand in hand. Sleep and mood exist in a bidirectional relationship—each exerts a significant influence over the other. They are both a symptom of depression and a trigger for the condition. Depression and sleep often exist in a debilitating cycle, each making the other worse. Insomnia is common among women (and men) who are depressed, and so is oversleeping or sleeping at the wrong times, which makes routine nighttime rest more difficult.

Stress is also a trigger for upsetting your sleep cycle. Our brains are unsettled, anxiety begins to rise, and, as a result, our circadian rhythms can be disrupted.

An essential step in taking care of your well-being is being proactive about your sleep habits and making sure that you get enough sound sleep. The importance of sleep cannot be overemphasized; sufficient sleep on a regular basis has the power to revitalize the brain, rebalance hormones, and restore your overall physiological, mental, and emotional functioning.

Stress: The Silent Menace

Stress is a major contributor to disease risk, weakening immune function and leaving you more vulnerable to getting sick. Stress is rampant in our society, and loss of estrogen makes you even more vulnerable to stress. Regardless of your present situation—married or single, caring for children or empty nester, managing a career or working part-time—you are more than likely trying to manage a full, demanding schedule. I can't bring to mind one patient of mine who does not have a constant, chronic amount of stress in her life. And although I cannot give advice on how to mitigate the individual sources of this stress, I can and do offer advice on how to better manage the stress so that it doesn't create disease and steal your health.

Oftentimes, my patients are not fully aware of the impact of stress on their physical and mental health. Indeed, the feeling of heightened tension, of the need for action and response under fire, can drain the body and mind of energy and wear down your immune system. Over time, this state of high alert—the physical manifestation of stress—erodes physiological health right down to the cellular level.

I know from firsthand experience the toll that stress can take. I used to work 120 hours a week in practice, never stopping, always exhausted, trying to meet and keep up with my family and professional demands. I, too, had to make meaningful changes to my lifestyle so that I could experience more balance and peace of mind. For you, this balance is of huge importance.

Stress causes a cascade of problems that undermines your ability to experience pleasure, to enjoy activities, relationships, and work. I think of stress as a sinister, very adept, and skillful thief: under the cloak of being productive and measuring up, stress steals your rest, joy, health, and vitality. At a biological level, stress interferes with hormone function and balance, diminishes cognitive function, and threatens the structural health of the brain. Stress exacerbates mood disorders, disrupts emotional balance and processing, and wears away at emotional resilience. To be blunt: stress ages you.

At a neurobiological level, stress is the consequence of the brain and body's response to perceived threat. That threat can be real (a car veering toward you in oncoming traffic) or perceived (the anticipation of a difficult conversation with your spouse). The brain-body knows no difference between actual threats and possible or perceived threats. Its response is the same, whether you are fretting while paying bills, nervously thinking about a job interview, or running from a bear. Whatever threat looms, the brain's hypothalamus signals the pituitary and adrenal glands to release the hormone cortisol. This hormone supplies you with heightened attention and vigilance, immediate energy to marshal a physical response—to fight or to flee. When this physiological response— designed to protect you from immediate and serious harm— occurs frequently enough, over time it damages the body at the cellular level. The damage affects every organ, every tissue, every physiological function—and makes you vastly more vulnerable to disease.

The exhaustion and depletion that results from stress leaves you increasingly vulnerable to more stress. Under chronic stress, your cortisol levels are consistently elevated and your adrenal glands are perpetually overworked. Eventually, the adrenal system stops functioning properly—it physically exhausts itself. At that point, the adrenal system can no longer operate at full, normal capacity, and the body has reached a condition of adrenal fatigue or exhaustion. Cortisol levels drop—the adrenal gland can no longer produce cortisol in abundance, even in response to highly stressful triggers. In a state of adrenal exhaustion, your energy levels plummet, you feel a deep and pervasive fatigue, and you have trouble functioning during the day and difficulty sleeping at night. A daily routine that once felt manageable and even enjoyable may now feel like an insurmountable effort. Severe adrenal depletion can, in rare cases, lead to Addison's disease, a life-threatening condition.

Estrogen is one of several hormones that, when in healthy, abundant supply, helps protect you from stress and its harmful consequences.

Cortisol: The Stress Hormone

Cortisol serves important metabolic and immunological functions, but, when chronically elevated, cortisol can cause physiological damage and increase risk for disease. Excessive cortisol

- Elevates blood pressure
- Causes cardiovascular damage
- Impairs immunity
- Triggers oxidative stress and inflammation
- Contributes to brain cell death, brain atrophy, and memory loss
- Exacerbates physical pain
- Doubles the risk of breast cancer

Migraines

Migraines and other forms of debilitating headaches occur more frequently among women than men. Women are three times more likely than men to experience migraines, and roughly 30 percent of women will suffer from one at some point in their lifetime. Migraine headaches are tremendously painful, often paralyzing, and temporarily disabling to normal life. Intense pressure, stabbing, and throbbing pain (in many cases localized to the temples) are often accompanied by nausea and vomiting, numbness in the extremities, and extreme sensitivity to light, sound, and smell. Many migraine sufferers experience visual disturbances, including flashing lights, blind spots, and blurred vision.

Levels of estrogen and other hormones are an important factor in a woman's risk of developing migraines. (Other significant factors are stress and lack of sleep, which are affected by both the presence of estrogen and estrogen deficiency.) When estrogen declines during the monthly cycle, you become more vulnerable to developing migraines or other severe, debilitating headaches. Once girls begin menstruating, they are more likely to get migraines. Migraines are most likely to occur in the week before your period, when estrogen is falling, and during menstruation, when estrogen is at its lowest. However, some women experience milder forms of migraines over the course of a month, when estrogen drops even slightly. Estrogen—specifically estradiol (E2)—acts as an anti-hyperalgesic, which means it lessens one's sensitivity to pain.

Progesterone can also be a factor in migraine onset for women. Falling progesterone and falling estrogen together can trigger migraines during the premenstrual week. Migraines that occur during menstruation itself are more likely to be the result of low estrogen.

For women with a history of migraine, pregnancy—with its soaring estrogens—can be a respite from these difficult headaches. But immediately after childbirth, a woman's body undergoes an abrupt, dramatic drop in estrogen, which can trigger a recurrence of migraines.

Perimenopause often brings an increase in migraines as a consequence of the irregular, often abrupt fluctuations of estrogen amid the hormone's overall decline. Migraines continue to be more frequent and severe for women during menopause itself. As menopause progresses and estrogen levels stabilize, the incidence of migraine may lessen and quiet.

Your Skeleton and Bones

Women are especially vulnerable to bone loss and osteoporosis as they age, and estrogen acts as an antioxidant and anti-inflammatory, playing a vital role in slowing bone loss. Estrogen and other hormone deficiencies increase your risk for osteoporosis. Women become more vulnerable to bone loss and osteoporosis during menopause, when estrogen levels decline. Women who use low-dose estrogen birth control are also at particular risk for bone loss and osteoporosis, since they have a perpetual deficit of estrogen. (The progestin-only birth control Depo-Provera is also a factor in osteoporosis.) Antidepressant SSRI medications contribute to the risk for osteoporosis; maintaining estrogen levels guards against depression and reduces the need for these medications. When you get into a state of chronic low estrogen, you are vulnerable to weakening bones and muscle tissue because estrogen helps maintain lean muscle mass and also helps in muscle healing.

Please keep in mind that many emotional or behavioral symptoms, such as anxiety, depression, or sleep disturbances, can have causes other than hormonal ones. The same is true for certain autoimmune illnesses, such as thyroid disorders (Graves' disease or Hashimoto's), osteopenia, diabetes, and cardiovascular disease, which have multiple causes that come together to wreak havoc on your body. Chronic stress, for instance, can have a cascade effect on multiple parts of your brain and body. These overlapping, interacting systems are exactly why I practice integrative medicine; by looking at your body and brain as a whole, I can more easily assess your underlying issues so that you can address problems directly. Your hormonal health is one way to understand how to both protect your health and ward off disease, but there are many other systems at play in preserving your brain and body wellness.

YOUR HEALTH JOURNAL: CHECK YOUR MEDICINE CABINET

This is a good time for you to take note of all your current medicines, as well as any other prescriptions—for antibiotics, for instance—that you have taken in the last twelve months. Make a list of these medicines in your journal, since it will be important information for your doctor to consider.

5

The Truth About Estrogen
and Breast Cancer

B reast cancer is the most common cancer in women. Each year in the United States, more than 200,000 women are diagnosed and more than 41,000 women die as a result of the disease. Currently, an American woman's lifetime risk of developing breast cancer is 12.4 percent—that's one out of every eight women. Yet more than one out of eight women fear breast cancer and believe they are at risk for developing it. In other words, most women overestimate their likelihood of developing breast cancer. Women also overestimate their family history and genetics as risk factors. And our ability to cure breast cancer has also improved dramatically. As Avrum Bluming, M.D., and Carol Tavris, Ph.D., point out clearly in their well-researched book *Estrogen Matters*, "In 2016, researchers calculated that localized breast cancer, the form found in the majority of newly diagnosed cases, has a five-year survival rate of 99 percent." And "by 2018 the cure rate for newly diagnosed breast cancer patients is 90 percent."

The good news is this: women have a lot of power to *lower* their risk of getting breast cancer, and they have a lot of power to *prevent* breast cancer from occurring. And though women tend to *under-estimate* this power over their risk factors, I want to reassure all of you again that you do not have to fear the use of estrogen: when used consistent with advice from your health care professionals, HRT does not cause breast cancer, HRT doesn't increase your risk of breast cancer, and HRT doesn't negatively interfere with breast-cancer treatments. Unfortunately, there are a lot of continued misconceptions about estrogen and its relationship to breast cancer. However, as world-renowned oncologist and professor at Hebrew University of Jerusalem Dr. Gershom Zajicek says quite clearly in his YouTube presentation, "Estrogen does not cause breast cancer." Two other leading physicians, citing their own work and the research of other prominent doctors, support this stance. Dr. O. Ylikorkala says the "refusal" to give women with breast cancer HRT is "not . . . supported by the observational data available so far on this question, because HRT has not increased the risk for breast-cancer recurrence. In fact, it is well established that HRT abolishes hot flushes and improves significantly these patients' quality of life." In a significant 1999 study, Brewster et al. showed that the concern that HRT might activate growth in occult metastatic sites and promote a rash of recurrences in breast cancer was *not confirmed.* And as Michael Baum, world-renowned breast cancer expert, states (as quoted by Bluming and Tavris, 2018), "I find it intolerable and inhuman that we should have to carry on in ignorance about the benefits and risks of prescribing hormone replacement therapy to women who have had breast cancer." Furthermore, Dr. W. T. Creasman, a prominent ob-gyn at Duke University, has said, "There seemed to be little if any risk in giving hormone replacement therapy to women who had breast cancer."

And finally, as Bluming and Tavris also reported, Henk Verheul, a Dutch oncologist, stated in his 2000 paper, "None of the current treatments for breast cancer—surgery, radiation, chemotherapy—

were negatively affected by estrogen." He and his colleagues concluded that "the prevalent opinion that estrogens and estrogen treatment are deleterious for breast cancer needs to be revisited." Multiple national and international studies on women with and without breast cancer confirm what I believe to be the absolute safety of HRT.

Indeed, recent studies have confirmed three significant findings:

- estrogen increases apoptosis, the mechanism for clearing out cancerous or precancerous cells
- estrogen reduces Maggiore pro-inflammation factor NFK beta, IL6, IL 11
- estrogen decreases breast cancer stem cells
- estrogen increases P53 factor, which protects against cancer

Why do I implore you to pay attention to these studies and others (listed at the back of the book)? Because I want to underscore my understanding of the safety of bioidentical estrogen. Three important studies have affirmed this point of view:

- In a 2006 study of 9,000 Japanese women, it was found that women who used HRT were less likely to develop breast cancer than women who did not use HRT.
- In a 2009 study, bioidentical HRT was shown to decrease the risk of breast cancer.
- In a 2002 study, women who used HRT showed a reduced risk of death from breast cancer compared with nonusers.

Like most diseases, breast cancer is complicated. And estrogen's relationship to breast cancer is also complex and, therefore, important to understand. Indeed, in this chapter I have chosen to address breast cancer not because other forms of cancer are unimportant but because breast cancer is so often misunderstood. I also want to share with you vital information not only about estrogen's role in causing or preventing breast cancer but also about how your behaviors—how you manage stress, what you eat, how frequently you exercise, and even your choice of clothes, cosmetics, and home products—can affect your potential for either avoiding this disease or making yourself more vulnerable to it.

It is not my intention to mesmerize or confuse you with data and statistics. However, I believe it's of the utmost importance that you have at your fingertips all the evidence of the safety of HRT. The following studies support the safety and protective benefits of HRT; please share with your physician.

Studies from basic research:

- Animals supplemented with Estradiol experienced a profound reduction in breast cancer tumor size. J The National Cancer Institute 2002 Aug; 94(15):1173. Jordan VK et al. Clin Cancer Res 2001; 7:3156–65. Joselyn VC et al.

- Mice given high doses of estrogen and progesterone at puberty reduced breast cancer by 60%, and eliminated HER-2. Breast Cancer Res 2007 Jan 26; 9(1): R12. Rajkumar L et al.

- Mice with breast similar to women's breast treated with bioidentical hormones showed significant reduction in breast cancer formation and progression. Breast Cancer Res 2007; 9(2):102. Jerry DJ.

- In one study, a group of mice with the same degree of breast cancer were put into two groups: one treated with standard aromatase inhibitor, the other with bioidentical estrogen. The outcome of the group treated with BI estrogen had longer, healthier lives and better survival rates.

Studies that show estrogen does not aggravate breast cancer

- Estradiol binds to Estrogen Receptor Beta that decreases breast cancer growth. Endocrinology 2006 Sep; 147(9):4132–50. Zhu BT et al.

- Estriol affects beta receptors that decrease breast tissue proliferation. Endocrinology 2006 Sep; 147(9):4132–50. Zhu BT et al. Endocrinology 2007; 148(2):538–547. Cvoro A et al.

- Estrogen suppresses invasion of ER+ breast cancer cells. In contrast to continued inaccurate suggestion that estrogen negatively impacts breast cancer stem cell, estrogen has a significant role in suppressing invasion through actin cytoskeletal remodeling. Nature communication 2018; 2980. Parker S et al.

- ERT after breast cancer treatment does not seem to increase a breast cancer event. J Clin Oncol 1999 May; 17(5): 1482–7. Vassilopoulou-Sellin R et al.

- Follow-up of women with breast cancer on HRT shows no increase of breast cancer death or recurrence. Arch Family Med. 1966 Jun; 5(6):341–8. Gambreal RD. Am J OB/GYN 1996 May; 174(5):1494–8. Disaia PJ et al.

- Lower risks of recurrence and mortality in women who used HRT after breast cancer diagnosis, than in women who did not. J Natl Cancer Inst 2001 May; 93(10):754–62. O'Meara ES et al.

- In a study group of 123 women (mean age, 65.4 +/– 8.85 years) who were diagnosed with breast cancer, including 69 patients who received estrogen replacement therapy for > or = 32 years after diagnosis, it was found that estrogen replacement therapy does not increase either the risk of recurrence or of death in patients with early breast cancer. These patients may be offered estrogen replacement therapy after a full explanation of the benefits, risks, and controversies. Am J Obstet Gynecol 2002 Aug; 187(2):289–94; discussion 294–5. Natarajan PK et al.

- Studies done in 2009 (Holtorf) and in 2011 (Files et al.) found that breast cancer treated by bioidentical HRT (including estradiol, progesterone, DHERA, and testosterone) showed superior outcomes compared to treatment by aromatase inhibitors.

Patricia and Isabelle: A Story of Two Sisters

When I first met Patricia and Isabelle, sisters three and a half years apart in age, they looked like twins. Their light brown hair was cut and styled the same way. Their hazel eyes were shaped very similarly. They were one inch in height and five pounds in weight apart. It was hard for me to tell which sister was fifty-two and which was fifty-five.

They came together, flying in from a city in the South, because they'd read about my bioidentical hormone treatments, which I believe are safe to use even for some women with family histories of breast cancer. Their mother had died from breast cancer the year before, and so they understandably did not want to take any chemicalized estrogen for their symptoms.

Patricia said, "I am sick and tired of feeling fuzzy-headed and not able to sleep. I'm married and want to stay that way. Can you help?"

"I certainly hope so," I said. I then asked Isabelle, "As the older sister, are your symptoms similar to your sister's?"

She blushed and said, "I'm the younger sister, and I think my symptoms are worse. I feel anxious and depressed."

In the end, it was only Patricia who let me treat her with a combination of bioidentical estrogen and progesterone. Isabelle resisted, unable to get past her fear that HRT would cause breast cancer, based on the old interpretations of the Women's Health Initiative report. I could see she was terrified, so I backed off.

I treated Patricia from afar, communicating a few times a year. After five years had passed, she came to see me in my office, accompanied by an older woman, who I thought must be an aunt or friend. But it was Isabelle, her younger sister. Isabelle's low estrogen had declined rapidly and caused a cascade of problems, including an early stage of breast cancer. These two lovely women experienced remarkably different paths of health and disease.

I share this story as a cautionary tale. You will learn a lot more about breast cancer and your own risks later in this chapter. But for now, I simply ask you to keep an open mind.

The Risks Associated with Your Reproductive History

There's no more striking illustration of how estrogen protects breast health than pregnancy. During pregnancy, all forms of estrogen increase substantially. Both estradiol (E2) and estrone (E1) increase by a factor of ten. Estriol (E3)—recognized scientifically as a powerful protector against breast cancer—rises by a factor of one thousand. Progesterone, human growth hormone (HGH), and testosterone also increase significantly. Together, these hormonal surges offer long-term protection against breast cancer; take a look at these statistics:

- Higher levels of estriol during pregnancy are associated with a 58 percent reduction in breast cancer incidence later in life.
- Women who become pregnant after developing breast cancer have significantly higher survival rates than women who do not become pregnant—98 percent compared to 80 percent, respectively. Studies show that even one pregnancy may

double a woman's chances of survival while also halving her chances of breast cancer recurrence.

- With each full-term pregnancy, a woman reduces her risk for breast cancer by 7 percent.
- Being pregnant as a young woman lowers breast cancer risk.
- Breast-feeding lowers the risk of breast cancer.

I witnessed this protective effect of pregnancy firsthand when I worked as a physician in an ethnically diverse community in Israel, where women largely followed a traditional lifestyle, which involved pregnancies that occurred every eighteen months to two years. These women exhibited very few of the conditions that we encounter in the United States and other modern industrialized societies and, instead, exhibited a low incidence of heart disease, diabetes, and obesity. They also had very low rates of breast cancer and gynecological cancers. It was also uncommon for the women I treated to experience PMS, headaches, cramping, irregular periods, abnormal bleeding, fibroids, or endometriosis—gynecological problems that are widespread in our society.

Please understand: I am not advocating for women to adopt a lifestyle that is focused on pregnancy and childbearing, spending years of their lives pregnant and breast-feeding and raising ten or more children. For most women today, this is neither desirable nor feasible. I use this example solely to illustrate estrogen's immense power as a protector of women's health.

Unfortunately, this positive association with pregnancy implies that never having been pregnant—known in scientific terms as nulliparity—increases the risk of all forms of breast cancer. Further, longer duration of menstruation is associated with a higher risk of breast cancer, as is early puberty and menstruation. Several factors that you are already familiar with are also involved in this early spike in estrogen, including being overweight and eating a diet high in sugar and saturated fat and processed foods. Weight gain and fat accumulation are both linked to the early onset of puberty and an increased risk of developing obesity.

Further aggravating this early rise in estrogen is the consumption of estrogenic foods, including genetically modified soy or soy-based foods, refined sugar, processed foods, and nonorganic meat and dairy. All these nonorganic, genetically modified foods contain up to twenty different types of chemicals and additives, many of which mimic estrogen in the body when consumed and act like xenoestrogens. The danger for girls is early onset of puberty; the risk for young women in childbearing years is a disruption in their ability to conceive, if that is their wish. And, again, the longer a woman menstruates, the greater the risk over time of developing breast cancer.

The Genetic Risks for Breast Cancer: A Minority

The two genetic variants most commonly associated with breast cancer, BRCA1 and BRCA2, are well understood in the medical community and have received a great deal of public attention, resulting in a high level of awareness among women about these genetic markers' connection to breast cancer and to ovarian and other gynecological cancers. These two genetic mutations significantly increase the likelihood for developing breast cancer. Compared with the 12.4 percent of women in the general population who will develop breast cancer, women with BRCA1 variation have a 45 percent risk of breast cancer, and women with BRCA2 have a 55–65 percent risk. However, having the BRCA1 or BRCA2 genetic variation does not mean with certainty that a woman will develop breast cancer or other gynecological cancers.

If you are not sure whether you carry the BRCA1 or BRCA2

gene, consider the following risk factors and consult your physician. I recommend seeking out genetic testing to see if you carry the BRCA 1 or BRCA 2 genes if you or a family member

- Has a known BRCA1 or BRCA2 mutation
- Is of Ashkenazi (Eastern European) Jewish ancestry
- had breast cancer diagnosed at a young age (premenopausal or younger than age fifty)
- has had triple negative breast cancer diagnosed at age sixty or younger
- has had breast cancer in both breasts (bilateral breast cancer)
- has had both breast and ovarian cancers
- has had ovarian cancer
- knows of a male relative with breast cancer

If any of the above applies to you, I also suggest that you speak with a genetic counselor to help you decide what other genetic testing options may be available based on your personal and family history.

However, these gene mutations are responsible for only a fraction of all breast cancer cases, accounting for somewhere between 5–10 percent of them. That means the overwhelming majority of breast cancers—at least 90 percent or more—originate from something other than BRCA1 or BRCA2 genetic factors.

Other genetic mutations that are less well known than the BRCA1 and BRCA2 gene variants but that affect a great many more women and increase their risk for breast cancer are single nucleotide polymorphisms, or SNPs, often referred to as "snips." Several different SNPs affect breast health and the likelihood of developing breast cancer, in some cases raising risks significantly. These genetic mutations influence the way women metabolize estrogen and also affect how vulnerable a woman is to other risk factors—particularly to environmental pollutants. Certain gene mutations affect genes that control how robustly and effectively a woman's body fends off the potential damage that chemical toxins can do to genes and cells that can lead to the development of breast cancer. Often, women with these SNPs have noticeable sensitivities to pollutants in the air, particularly those that arise from the burning of substances—exhaust from cars, tobacco smoke, smoke from a fire or a barbecue. Pay attention to these sensitivities if you have them and take steps to avoid exposure to these pollutants. A number of genetic tests can tell you if you have SNPs and also alert you to the presence of potentially harmful estrogen metabolites. Again, if you are at all concerned that you may have a genetic vulnerability, speak to your physician about genetic testing.

Depression and Breast Cancer

Depression increases the risk of developing a broad array of diseases, including breast cancer. Depression dampens immune function, slows treatment recovery time, and impedes healing. Major depression is associated with a 380 percent increase in the risk of breast cancer. To complicate matters further, many women with breast cancer feel depressed and are then put on antidepression medications such as an SSRI, which has been shown to increase the formations of both estrogen receptor and progesterone receptor tumors. In at least one study, the SSRI paroxetine was associated with a 720 percent increase in breast cancer. However, women are often given SSRIs during standard breast cancer treatment, which has been shown to increase deaths from breast cancer by 75 percent.

How Your Lifestyle Can Reduce or Increase Your Risk

Some of the most underappreciated factors that contribute to breast cancer risk are related to your lifestyle—what you eat, how regularly you exercise, and how you manage stress. By eating well, exercising sufficiently, and making sure that your stress-busting techniques are working for you, you can not only sustain your hormonal balance but also protect yourself from developing breast cancer. In upcoming chapters, I will explain the many choices available to you—diet and supplements, exercise, stress management, and other daily actions—that can help you lower your risk for breast cancer and become healthier overall. Here, we will look at several lifestyle choices that are associated with an elevated breast cancer risk.

Weight and Diet

Being overweight or obese and gaining significant weight during adulthood can substantially raise your risk for breast cancer. Many studies have demonstrated this effect. A woman is at greater risk for breast cancer if she gains

- More than 55 pounds in her adult lifetime
- More than 22 pounds after menopause
- 38 pounds or more during pregnancy (This weight gain in pregnancy not only elevates the risk for the mother, but also increases her unborn daughter's risk of developing breast cancer.)

Beyond its effects on weight gain, diet is also an important risk factor for breast cancer. A diet heavy in processed foods—that is, foods high in sugar and "bad" fats—puts women at higher risk for the disease. So does a diet that routinely includes red meat.

As you consider these statistics, keep in mind these are not meant to scare you but to help motivate you to reconsider how you eat.

- The typical Western diet is associated with a 45 percent elevation in breast cancer risk.
- Foods high in omega-6 fat—an unhealthful fat found in corn oil and common in processed foods—significantly elevates breast cancer risk. A diet that regularly includes omega-6 fats contributes to a more than 100 percent increase in breast cancer risk.
- A diet high in dairy products increases the likelihood of developing breast cancer.
- Eating 1.5 servings of red meat daily results in a 97 percent increase in breast cancer.
- Women in the top 25 percent of sugar intake have twice the risk of breast cancer as those who consume the least sugar. A high-sugar diet raises breast cancer risk by 63 percent.
- Women who are the highest bread consumers have a 28 percent greater risk of developing breast cancer than women who are the lowest bread consumers.

In short, a high-calorie, low-nutrient diet and a sedentary lifestyle will put you on a road to problems with your metabolism, which in turn contribute to increased risk for breast cancer. High glucose (blood sugar) levels (from a diet heavy in sugar and starchy foods) have a strong association with breast cancer and also have been scientifically shown to interfere with the effectiveness of chemotherapy in eradicating breast cancer cells. Insulin resistance, the metabolic disorder that stems from chronically high blood sugar, is linked to a 210 percent increase in certain breast cancer tumors. Women who develop metabolic syndrome—a condition that includes a cluster of symptoms involving weight, poor cardiovascular health, and unhealthful blood glucose levels—have a greater chance both of developing breast cancer and of dying from the disease. The presence of metabolic syndrome in women over sixty increases their risk of dying from breast cancer by 23 percent. For women of all ages, metabolic syndrome increases the risk of developing breast cancer by 52 percent, and research has found that women with breast cancer are more likely to have metabolic syndrome. Elevated cholesterol also raises the risk of breast cancer. A metabolite (by-product) of cholesterol acts like estrogen in a woman's body and can encourage growth of breast cancer cells, causing breast cancer to be more aggressive.

- The intestinal disorder known as leaky gut syndrome can increase breast cancer risk. With leaky gut syndrome, the intestinal barrier weakens and triggers inflammation, which can cause breast cancer as well as other diseases. The weakened intestinal barrier also allows the spread of cancer-causing substances throughout the body.
- Smoking increases risks for many cancers, including breast cancer. Current smokers carry a 16 percent greater risk of breast cancer than nonsmokers. For women who have other factors that elevate their breast cancer risk, smoking is particularly harmful, raising their risks by an additional 30 percent. Women who smoke a pack a day for more than a decade are especially at risk for the most common form of breast cancer.

Sleep and Stress

Insufficient sleep has been shown to contribute to the development of more aggressive breast cancers. Sleep apnea—a form of sleep-disordered breathing that causes interruptions to normal breath flow during sleep—increases a woman's risk of breast cancer by more than 100 percent. Sleep apnea is often regarded as a male sleep disorder, but it affects women as well, and women are at particular risk for going undiagnosed. Disruptions to normal circadian function—the body's twenty-four-hour sleep-wake cycle— have been linked to increased risk for breast cancer. Women who have frequent night shifts at work, where the risks for circadian disruption are high, have a high risk for breast cancer. Research shows that female nurses who worked more than five years of six consecutive night shifts saw an 80 percent increase in their breast cancer risk. Recently sleep apnea has been found to increase the risk of breast cancer in women, in part due to the weight gain some women experience in menopause.

Stress compromises the immune system, triggers inflammation, and exposes women to greater risk for breast cancer. Stress increases the circulating tumor cell marker AGR2 and contributes to increased risk of metastasis.

Medications Associated with Breast Cancer Risk

Millions of women regularly use medications for health conditions that, unbeknownst to them, raise their risks for breast cancer. It's important to be fully informed about the risks associated with the medications you take. An integrative medical doctor will be more informed than a physician who practices strictly Western medicine about the negative side effects of certain medicines and their interactions with cancer-causing triggers.

The use of antibiotics over a woman's lifetime is a factor in her breast cancer risk. Indeed, the use of antibiotics for 51–100 days over a lifetime is associated with a 53 percent increase in the risk of breast cancer. Lifetime antibiotic use between 501 and 1,000 days results in a 114 percent increase in breast cancer risk.

In addition, women who use sedative medicines, such as Ambien for sleep and Valium or Xanax for anxiety, can elevate their risk for breast cancer. In one study, taking eighteen pills or more per year was associated with an increased risk for breast cancer and a higher overall mortality rate.

And, as mentioned above, SSRIs, a group of medications commonly used to treat depression and anxiety, have also been shown to raise the risk for breast cancer, especially for women already in menopause.

Statin drugs, which are used to lower cholesterol, can also significantly increase the risk of developing an aggressive form of breast cancer, as well as diabetes. Other medications that are widely used in the treatment of cardiovascular disease also lead to higher risks for breast cancer, including ACE inhibitors, which treat blood pressure, and calcium channel blockers, also used for high blood pressure. Women who spend more than five years taking high blood pressure medication face greater risks for an estrogen-positive form of invasive breast cancer. Digoxin, a medication that treats irregular heart rhythms, including atrial fibrillation, has also been shown in at least one study to increase breast cancer risk among current users. (This elevated risk does not appear to extend to former users.)

Breast cancer does not develop overnight. I sometimes ask my patients how long they think cancer cells must grow within a breast before the growth reaches a point where it can be picked up during a breast exam. Most women estimate somewhere between a few months to a few years. My patients are surprised to learn—as you also may be—that cancer takes much, much longer than that to grow. From the time of a first cell mutation to when a growth can be felt takes an average of fifteen years. This means, among other things, that you have time to influence your risk for breast cancer and how that cancer does—or does not—develop.

How You Can Help to Avoid Breast Cancer

We know a lot about cancer. We know that the body's immune system fights off most cancers before they have a chance to develop. We know that certain lifestyle choices increase or decrease one's chances for developing cancer. We know that certain genes increase one's vulnerability to cancer. We know that it takes at least five to six mutations (even in the presence of carcinogens) for any cell to become cancerous. So though there is no guarantee that you won't develop cancer—in particular, breast cancer—understanding how cancer is triggered is a very good first step to reducing your risk and possibly preventing cancer from ever taking root.

Keeping in mind that it takes, on average, fifteen years for cancer to develop, we should want to take any precaution necessary to avoid triggering mutation. What does this mean in terms of breast cancer in particular?

1. Eat a diet full of vegetables that contain phytonutrients, which act as antioxidants and fight off free radicals that may try to mutate a cell.
2. Exercise, sweat, and otherwise boost your body's ability to eliminate bad cells.
3. Keep your gut healthy with probiotics and a clean diet; the gut is, in many ways, the center of our immune system since it manages the elimination of extra foods our body does not need.
4. Reduce your exposure to chemicals in foods, cosmetics, household

products, clothing, and furnishings that can trigger cell mutations.

5. Consider taking a daily dose of Alka Seltzer Gold, which contains
   bicarbonate and is a well-established anti-inflammatory that can
   help prevent autoimmune disease and cancer.

6. Add the supplement low-dose naltrexone (LDN—in a 1.5–4.5 mg
   dosage range) to support the immune system; LDN also acts as
   an anti-inflammatory, antiviral, and antibacterial agent.

You will read more about these steps in the diet and exercise
chapters later in the book.

When Considering Diagnosis and Treatment

This year many women will receive a diagnosis of breast cancer
and begin the arduous, frightening, often confusing pursuit of
treatment. Today, medical doctors, researchers, and others have
made a lot of progress when it comes to the treatment of this once
fatal disease. I want you to understand the landscape of prevention
and treatment options, some of which will help you recover faster
and better, so that you can get the support you need during any
stage of this process.

The current conventional approach to breast cancer treatment is often anti-estrogen. Estrogen—the single most important hormone to women's health, the original breast cancer
fighter—has become enemy number one in the current climate
of breast cancer therapy. I'm hoping that a more complete and
accurate understanding of estrogen's health-enhancing role in
both preventing and treating breast cancer will soon become
more widely known and acknowledged, so that you can feel

more hopeful and empowered if you ever do receive a diagnosis of breast cancer.

The Pros and Cons of Mammograms

In 2009, the United States Preventive Services Task Force, or USPSTF, made significant changes to its mammography screening recommendations, recommending against it for women ages 40–49. The task force recommended biannual—not yearly—screening mammograms for women ages 50–74. These new recommendations caused an uproar. Media coverage was skeptical and fearful, demonstrating significant bias against these changed recommendations without, for the most part, delving into the scientific evidence that led to the changes. The USPSTF itself also was at fault, failing to do enough to make the recommendations and their scientific context clear—to women directly or to the media, It was a wasted opportunity to educate the public about the limited usefulness and serious risks associated with mammography.

The revised recommendations put the task force at odds with some (but not all) breast cancer and women's health advocacy groups. Several were vehemently against the changes and remain so. Others—including the National Breast Cancer Coalition, Breast Cancer Action, and the National Women's Health Network—supported and welcomed the new guidelines, which, if followed, would result in fewer mammograms for most women over the course of their lifetime. They were right to do so.

The steps taken by the USPSTF are an instance of policy coming closer into alignment with scientific evidence. For instance, consider these study results:

- A Norwegian study found mammography screening saved 2.4 lives per 100,000 women screened.

- Mammography at age fifty leads to a benefit for only 1 out of 1,000 women.
- There is minimal to no reduction in the incidence of late-stage cancers in women who receive mammograms, compared to those who do not. Regular mammography results in a barely perceptible change in the diagnosis of these advanced, often aggressive, forms of the disease.
- Mammography screening results in almost no change to the survival rates for women with breast cancer.
- For older women, women with a projected life span of less than ten years, research indicates the risks of cancer are too slight to warrant mammograms.

Breast density is its own risk factor for breast cancer, and for contralateral breast cancer—a relatively rare metastasis of cancer in the second breast. Women in the top 25 percent of mammographic density are five times more likely to develop breast cancer. However, breast density does not affect women's mortality risks from breast cancer. The chemicalized hormones estrogen and progesterone together promote breast density, as does chemicalized progesterone by itself. (On its own, chemicalized estrogen does not increase breast density.)

Maternal characteristics appear to play a role in the development of dense breast tissue: women born to older mothers, age thirty-nine and over, are more likely to have dense breasts. So too are women who were relatively tall and thin before they underwent puberty. Dietary habits can also increase the likelihood of developing dense breasts: a high-fat diet, a diet high in red meat consumption, and alcohol consumption are all associated with the development of dense breast tissue. Dense breast tissue also makes it difficult to detect breast cancer, making mammograms less effective for screening and picking up early signs of breast cancer.

The earlier that mammography screening begins, the more likely women are to experience false-positive results. False-positive results are 60 percent more common in women who begin mammography screening at age forty. Research indicates that a third or more of mammography screenings will return abnormal results that ultimately do not correspond to actual cancer.

Estimates indicate that over the past thirty years more than one million women in the United States have been diagnosed with breast cancer that would have proved nonfatal if left undetected and untreated. What other health problems have those women suffered as a result of the invasive and toxic procedures used to diagnose and/or treat cancers that would have been okay to be left alone? Figures vary, but the estimates of overdiagnosis of breast cancer hover in the range of 20 to 30 percent of all breast cancers diagnosed. This is no small or isolated problem. Overdiagnosis of breast cancer is estimated to cost about a billion dollars annually.

BRCA1 and BRCA2 Are Special Cases

If you have BRCA1 or BRCA2, you are in a different treatment category than are women without these genetic markers. If you have inherited either of these gene mutations, you need to take special care and act as quickly as possible after a diagnosis, which often means surgery, a single mastectomy, or double mastectomies. These women are heroic in their courage to take the step of surgery. And with the sophistication of modern reconstructive surgery, many women, including some of my own patients, are very happy with their new breasts.

Another concerning genetic marker for cancer is the KRAS-variant, a biologically functional, microRNA-binding site variant that is associated with recurrent breast and ovarian cancer, lung and pancreatic cancer, and head and neck cancer. The KRAS-variant is often overlooked, despite its being very common—on average, one in twenty people carry this biomarker and one in four people with cancer show this genetic variation. Researchers have found that when patients with KRAS-variant discontinue hormone replacement therapy, there is an increased risk of triple negative breast cancer. In addition, KRAS-variant breast cancer patients had greater than an eleven-fold increased risk of presenting with MPBC (multiple primary breast cancer) compared to nonvariant patients (45.39 percent versus 6.78 percent). Thus, estrogen withdrawal and a low estrogen state appear to increase breast cancer risk and predict aggressive tumor biology in women with the KRAS-variant.

Anti-Estrogen Cancer Medicines

Before tamoxifen was discovered in 1966, most women with breast cancer were treated with estrogen, a synthetic version of estradiol (E2). And today, when anti-estrogen medications stop working, physicians often return to very high doses of estrogen to jump-start treatment—again, this points to the ultimate safety and benefit of treating breast cancer with estrogen. Recent studies have shown both the safety and effectiveness of estrogen for preventing and healing breast cancer. Specifically, estradiol has been used to bind with estrogen receptor cells and thereby decrease breast cancer growth, and estriol is used to target estrogen beta-receptors, which also decrease breast tissue proliferation.

Tamoxifen

Tamoxifen is probably the most well-known breast cancer medication. It functions by binding with estrogen receptors, thereby short-circuiting the cancer from developing or spreading. However, though tamoxifen can cut off cancer's ability to grow, the medicine does pose some serious side effects. If your oncologist recommends tamoxifen, discuss the possible side effects that include the following:

- At least one study showed an increased cancer recurrence of 440 percent for ER negative cancers
- Negative effect on eyesight
- Promotes cell invasion in breast cancer cells, even spurring tumor growth
- May turn the immune system away from fighting breast cancer cells, allowing those cells to grow unchecked
- Increases risk of uterine cancer
- Elevates risk for stroke
- Increases risk for deep vein thrombosis and pulmonary embolism

Aromatase Inhibitors

Aromatase inhibitors (AIs) are a class of drugs used to treat breast cancer and ovarian cancer in postmenopausal women. They disable the conversion of androgens to estrogen. Like tamoxifen, these drugs can cause problems with cognition and memory, as well as cardiovascular problems and deterioration of bone health. In addition, aromatase inhibitors increase expression of a protein (HER2/neu) that is an important biomarker for breast cancer, which can contribute to the growth and aggressiveness of breast cancer, ovarian cancer, and endometrial cancer. The presence of this protein is linked to higher rates of recurrence.

Again, if your oncologist recommends AIs, I encourage you to ask about the possible side effects, which include

- Cognitive dysfunction, inducing problems with memory and learning
- Increased risk of osteoarthritis
- Increased vulnerability to bone fractures
- Carpal tunnel syndrome
- Slow wound healing
- Sexual dysfunction (during active treatment)

One particular side effect of AIs is aromatase inhibitor musculo-skeletal syndrome, or AIMSS, which is often a disabling condition that has been found to occur in approximately half of women who take aromatase inhibitors. Caused by the estrogen deficiency these drugs induce, AIMSS causes widespread pain, stiffness, and swelling at joints throughout the body, often in the hands, wrists, ankles, and feet. AIMSS causes pain and restriction to movement and flexibility and is frequently treated with opioids, drugs that themselves can promote tumor growth and the spread of cancer.

But I do urge caution here. You should always get a second and even a third opinion to gain a complete understanding of your own individual situation and the risks involved. Breast cancer, thankfully, is becoming more of a chronic disease requiring long-term management instead of one that is always life-threatening. As you consider your own genetic, lifestyle, and other risks, I hope that you can keep in mind the limitations and dangers that arise from some of the established treatments described here. Even scientists who study the efficacy of cancer treatment reveal their own bias in reporting accurately on the limitations and dangers associated with chemotherapy and radiation. For instance, scientists tend to underreport the limits of usefulness and the toxicity of treatments for breast cancer by putting the information in less visible places in their reports. As a result, physicians and their patients don't get a complete picture.

YOUR HEALTH JOURNAL: WHAT ARE *YOUR* RISKS?

Although I do not want you to fall into a well of fear about developing breast cancer, it is important that you consider any of the risk factors related to your genetic heritability (especially for BRCA1 and BRCA2, as well as KRAS-variant), your lifestyle (including your diet), and other health issues that may increase your vulnerability. Remember, cancer takes a long time to develop; your body comes with its own layers of protection—you have the power to strengthen these protections and lessen your overall risk of disease.

Part Three

. . . .

Getting What You Need
for Your Best Self

6

Pulling It All Together

Estrogen affects every aspect of a woman's identity—and it affects each woman differently. Each woman has different signs and symptoms of estrogen deficiency, estrogen-progesterone imbalance, deficient testosterone, or other hormonal irregularities. Your need may be very different from that of your sister or best friend. So your next step is to establish whether you have low estrogen levels—or an estrogen deficiency—by getting tested. You need to find a physician who is knowledgeable and open to bioidentical hormone treatment, who is interested in listening to you and working with you. I suggest that you find a doctor or health care provider who is trained in integrative medicine; like me, these doctors tend to think of treatment holistically. Thousands of these doctors have been prescribing bioidentical treatment for years, and they have had the same success with patients that I have had.

Taking Next Steps: Your Hormonal Profile

You are the expert on your feelings and symptoms. No physician or test can match your familiarity, your insight, your instincts about how you feel, what changes have occurred in your life physically, mentally, and emotionally. This is why I've asked you to keep notes in your health journal throughout the course of this book. These notes and lists of symptoms and other relevant details will help your physician understand your body's production of estrogen and its effects, your symptoms of estrogen deficiency or excess. Keep in mind that it is never too late to consider hormone replacement therapy (HRT). If, for instance, you were part of the fear wave after the Women's Health Initiative study and stopped HRT, you can absolutely begin to supplement again. If you've been on synthetic hormones and wish to move to bioidentical HRT, all you need to consider is to give your body time for the synthetic chemicals to leave your body. (It typically takes six weeks for Premarin to leave your system; for progestin it's typically quicker. In both cases, you will need to take your blood measurements to get an accurate assessment of your various hormone levels.)

Any woman—regardless of where she is on the perimenopause-menopause continuum—can benefit from HRT. In some cases, if a woman is past fifty-six years old, the effectiveness of HRT may not be as robust; however, she can still benefit from estrogen, progesterone, and testosterone—especially if she wants to live a more energetic, sexually active, and otherwise vibrant life.

Review Your Health History

As you ready yourself to find a physician and decide on the hormone tests you may need, ask yourself the questions in the health history review that follows.

What can you recall about puberty and your personal
   transition from girl to woman?
How did the developmental changes to your body affect
   you mentally, physically, emotionally?
What were your periods like during adolescence: regular,
   light, heavy, irregular?
Did you have PMS symptoms?

Now reflect on your young adulthood and reproductive years:

What pattern does your monthly cycle follow, or what
   patterns did it follow? Was your cycle long or brief,
   regular or irregular?
Did you have symptoms of PMS or other symptoms of low
   or excess estrogen during your monthly cycle, such as low
   mood, anxiety, irritability, or bad cramps? How intense
   were they? When did they occur? Did they differ from the
   symptoms you had as an adolescent, if you had PMS then?
What is or was perimenopause like? What physical and
   emotional symptoms, such as changes in mood or sleep
   patterns that may be related to estrogen decline, can you
   identify?

If you are in menopause, consider what symptoms you have
that indicate estrogen fluctuations and signs of estrogen decline.

When did menopause begin?
How intense are your symptoms? Are they physical,
   mental, emotional? Which symptoms have been most
   difficult or intrusive?

Identify all symptoms and their frequency.

• • •

By walking yourself through all the stages of your life, up to the present, you'll gradually paint a picture of an estrogen history that is yours alone. This information will be invaluable to you and your physician as you explore bioidentical estrogen and other bioidentical hormone supplements. These details and this insight provide you with important clues about how much estrogen your body needs to feel normal—your normal, not anyone else's.

For this reason, when it comes to measuring estrogen levels and assessing a "need" for estrogen therapy, there really is no firm, fixed definition of "normal." There exists a range of estrogen that is considered a technical, official normal range for estrogen levels in the blood. But blood estrogen levels don't tell the whole story. For many women, their true, natural, unique estrogen "normal" level falls outside that general range—because that's how their bodies work. A woman with high natural estrogen may test within the normal range on an estrogen blood test and yet be experiencing significant signs and effects of estrogen deficiency. A woman with low natural estrogen may display symptoms of estrogen excess before even crossing the lower threshold of the normal range. One woman's high estrogen will be another woman's low. The true picture of a woman's estrogen need depends on what her body naturally produces and how her body responds to estrogen fluctuations and declines.

Remember, you may not have symptoms all the time, and your symptoms may fluctuate. For instance, you may not be in perimenopause but still may be in a low-estrogen or estrogen-deficiency state.

Finding the Right Physician

The best physician is a partner in all aspects of your health, including your hormonal health and balance. When choosing a physician, consider the following:

Knowledge and expertise. Ideally, your physician has experience in preventive medicine as well as working with bioidentical hormones. Finding physicians familiar with and open to using bioidentical estrogen and other bioidentical hormones is not as difficult as it used to be, as more of the medical establishment recognizes the differences between chemicalized hormone supplements and bioidentical hormone supplements.

Time. It takes time to manage bioidentical hormone therapy effectively and well. You need regular check-ins, communications about changing symptoms, and alterations of dosage as needs and hormone levels change. Too many physicians unfortunately remain locked in a schedule that's dehumanizing for both doctor and patient, with patients pushed through doctors' offices and examination rooms on assembly-line timetables.

An open mind. The right physician is willing to educate her- or himself about new and emerging techniques and to listen carefully to her or his patient's interests, hopes, and desires.

A life-promoting outlook. A physician works not only to prevent disease but also to enhance your life. Does your physician offer nutrition and other lifestyle counseling? Physicians and practitioners who are trained in an integrative approach will incorporate these health recommendations into any counseling or discussions of next steps.

If your current physician does not share these attributes, you may not need to switch doctors if he or she is interested in learning about bioidentical estrogen therapy and exploring their use. The first step is to express your interest to your physician and ask if he or she can work with you.

If you do find yourself looking for a physician who works with bioidentical hormones, a first step might be to take a look at the provider list of the American Association of Integrative Medicine (www.aaimedicine.com/fap/). I've listed other helpful resources at the back of the book. Your physician will more than likely already have a relationship with a local and trustworthy compounding pharmacy to source your hormonal therapy supplements. However, as a general rule of thumb, the best source of compounding pharmacies is the Pharmacy Compounding Accreditation Board (PCAB), which is a service of the national Accreditation Commission for Health Care. PCAB-accredited pharmacies can add a great deal of peace of mind. This doesn't mean a nonaccredited pharmacy is not providing high-quality or safe products as well, but you should research where your compounded bioidentical hormones are made and the rigor of the safety protocols and standards used to make them.

Tests Before Beginning Bioidentical HRT

Before beginning any hormone therapy, you should have a full physical and gynecological exam in order to make sure that you have healthy levels of other hormones, especially thyroid hormones, cortisol (the hormone that is produced in response to stress), and insulin (the hormone that regulates blood sugar). These hormones need to be in a healthy range before you begin taking bioidentical hormones, including estrogen, progesterone, and others. (See below for specific tests related to cortisol, insulin, and thyroid hormones).

You also want to begin to follow a clean diet that is rich in fiber, greens, protein, and quality dietary fats. This will help your body maximize its response to HRT and will also help you think about this next phase of your life as a lifestyle change.

As you read through the information about tests below, keep your journal handy so that you can make a list of the tests that you think you need and questions that you have about them. Refer to this list when you meet with your physician, so that you remember to ask all your questions. You can also use your journal to keep track of your test results and to make notes about what those results mean, what deficiencies they show, and how your doctor recommends that you remedy them.

There are three basic hormone test types that can be done to assess your various hormone levels:

Blood Serum/Plasma

Testing your blood serum is generally accepted to be the most reliable test to measure hormone levels and is often covered by insurance. I use this test 98 percent of the time because it is particularly good at measuring levels of LH, FSH, prolactin, fasting insulin, and thyroid hormones, including reverse T3 and thyroid antibodies. It is also used to measure sex hormone–binding globulin (SHBG) and, less commonly, cortisol-binding globulin (CBG). However, since only the serum is measured, the serum test is not as helpful for testing sex hormone because estradiol, estrone, and estriol (the three major estrogens) and progesterone are measured as totals of both bound and free hormones; the test does not break down specific amounts of each. Relying on these totals may lead to inaccurate measures of your discreet hormone levels. For example, it may appear that your hormone level is normal or high because of an abundance of a bound hormone. This may be hiding the fact that your free hormone level is actually low.

The blood serum test is also limited in that it only gives a snapshot of your hormone levels at one point on one day. Hormone levels fluctuate throughout the day and week, and it's often unclear whether the levels reflect a low or high point in the day.

Saliva

Many doctors, including me, sometimes use saliva tests to measure free-form hormones in the body. However, your physician should have access to sophisticated lab technology to make sure samples are not tainted (by gum disease, for instance). Also, if you are menopausal and you suspect you have very low levels of estrogen and/or progesterone, your hormone levels might not be detectable in a saliva sample. Saliva tests are simple, convenient take-home tests, but they are not covered by many insurance companies and can be expensive.

Urine

Urine tests can give accurate readings of hormone levels. Although a urine test can give you an accurate reading of one day, it will not show variations over the course of several days. Urine tests are not as convenient as saliva and require a visit to the lab or doctor's office, but they are not expensive.

Of these three types of tests, none alone is optimal. Saliva works well when you have not yet taken any hormones. But once you start taking hormones and you're checking for optimal levels, saliva becomes less reliable because levels go up so quickly; and there is very little correlation between levels and how you actually feel. The newer urine test may have some benefit in showing estrogen metabolism, where your hormones are coming from, and where they are going. However, I mainly rely on serum blood tests as a starting point. Then, as I hear back from my patients about how they feel as they begin a supplementation program, I retest them until we figure out the optimal amounts (dosages) and balance of the hormones.

Assessing Your Estrogen Levels

When assessing your overall hormone levels, a full-screen blood serum test can be used to measure a number of different hormones.

ESTRADIOL (E2)

You will begin with the estradiol (E2) blood test. This test establishes a baseline blood estrogen level. If you have been using chemicalized estrogen or other chemicalized hormone replacement, results of an estradiol blood test will not be accurate for at least eight weeks after you stop taking these hormone substitutes.

Also, ask to include three other important hormone measurements, including

SHBG

This test of sex hormone–binding globulin levels provides a more comprehensive portrait of estrogen levels.

FSH

Measuring FSH (follicle-stimulating hormone) levels will help indicate whether your estrogen symptoms are related to perimenopause or menopause. When it's high, you should test free estradiol because your level may be high; normal estrogen ranges from -4.7 to 21.5 mIU/mL. When a woman has not had a period for over a year and her FSH level is consistent at 100 mIU/mL, it's usually an indication that she is in menopause.

Estrogen Metabolism

If you or someone in your family has had breast cancer, it's also important to test for estrogen metabolism (how well your body breaks down and eliminates excess estrogen). Estrogen-metabolism testing measures the levels of three different estrogen metabolites, which are products of the body's use of estrogen, including 2-hydroxy estrone; 16-hydroxy estrone; and 4-hydroxy estrone. The metabolite 2-hydroxy estrone protects against breast cancer, while the remaining two estrogen metabolites can signal an increased risk for breast cancer. Measuring the levels of these individual metabolites as well as the ratio of 2-hydroxy estrone to 16-hydroxy estrone and 4-hydroxy estrone can provide information about individual breast cancer risk.

Assessing Progesterone Levels

How you feel is an important factor in determining your need for progesterone, but, again, a blood test will reveal the level most accurately. There is a range of progesterone in your blood that is generally optimal, and many physicians and laboratories use the range of 15–25 ng/mL as an indicator of the normal range. However, I use a narrower range of 18–20 ng/mL because I find that many women are very sensitive to low progesterone.

If you are still menstruating, the ideal time to test for progesterone is during the week before your period, when your progesterone is at its peak. If you are in perimenopause or menopause and you recognize signs of low progesterone, such as increased irritability and difficulty sleeping, you can test anytime to get a more accurate reading of your levels. Progesterone usually declines as the ovaries decrease their production of it and as other hormones fluctuate. I recommend that women of any age supplement with progesterone to restore a feeling of calm and relaxation.

Assessing Testosterone Levels

One of the most misunderstood hormone measurements is testosterone. Measuring the blood level of testosterone is almost meaningless because it does not capture how much testosterone is in the cell. As you've seen, in principle, any woman in menopause moves from an estrogen-dominant environment to one dominant in testosterone. I always ask if she is feeling aggressive, growing hair on her chin, losing hair on her head, and developing acne; if she says yes, I give her estrogen.

To assess your testosterone levels, you need two measurements: a total testosterone level and a free testosterone level. The range of "normal" total testosterone is generally between 30–80 ng/dL. But this can vary individually. Women who are muscular may naturally have a higher level, while women without as much muscle may have a lower level but still be in balance. Free testosterone is the amount of testosterone that's available for the body to use; it also reflects the SHBG levels and, indirectly, estrogen levels. Remember, estrogen increases levels of sex hormone–binding globulin.

A serum blood test is the best way to measure testosterone levels accurately. Any supplementation should be done in small doses so that the optimal level is reached gradually. Paying attention to how you feel as you take the supplements is critical so that you find the right balance of dosage. How a woman feels is equally critical to balancing testosterone. The goal should be to alleviate problems associated with testosterone levels that are too low and to take advantage of the benefits of supplemental testosterone without creating side effects or signs of excess.

Assessing Human Growth Hormone (HGH) Levels

The most accurate way to measure HGH is actually through measuring IGF-1 (insulin-like growth factor), a biochemical made by the liver in response to HGH. With HGH, the standard "normal" blood levels aren't applicable to all women. Therefore, a blood test measuring HGH isn't the definitive answer to whether HGH is needed. Again, assessing whether your HGH levels are low to see if you may benefit from HGH supplementation begins with identifying possible related symptoms. I also recommend that you get these other tests before taking HGH, which most physicians also recommend:

Lipids
CBC (complete blood count)
C-reactive protein
Thyroid function
Insulin
Hemoglobin A1C
Glucose
Testosterone
Cortisol
Insulin-like growth factor 1
Insulin-like growth factor binding protein 3

Assessing Cortisol Levels

The main function of the hormone cortisol, which is produced by the adrenal glands, is to help manage the brain and body's response to stress. It also helps manage how our bodies break down carbohydrates, fats, and proteins. Too much chronic high cortisol not only can deplete your body's adrenal glands (cause adrenal fatigue, for instance) but also can cause Cushing's syndrome (too much cortisol, often from steroid medications for asthma, rheumatoid arthritis, and lupus). When you have chronically low cortisol, you can develop a very rare condition called Addison's disease (or primary adrenal insufficiency, when the body does not produce enough cortisol). Along with checking your other hormones, it's important to understand your cortisol levels as a way to monitor your brain-body's ability to manage stress. Your cortisol blood level can be measured in three ways: through your blood, saliva, or urine.

Assessing DHEA Levels

A deficiency of DHEA doesn't manifest with symptoms as do deficiencies of other hormones. To measure DHEA, I recommend testing blood for DHEAS (DHEA-sulfate). These levels are at their peak in your twenties, when a normal range is 500–3,000 ng/mL or 50–300 ug/dL. As we age, DHEA and other hormone levels diminish significantly. By your fifties, you can expect to have lost roughly 70 percent of your natural DHEA supply. Replacing DHEA is about finding the point at which your body is benefiting from the supplement without side effects.

Assessing Pregnenolone Levels

In general, I have noticed a trend toward very low levels of pregnenolone—in the young and old. Although pregnenolone levels decline with age, it's important to measure pregnenolone when you're doing a regular blood serum test to make sure you have an optimal level. Pregnenolone assists in protecting against symptoms of aging, and it seems to have a balancing effect on other hormones, naturally adjusting their levels up or down. For normal steroid hormone production, cholesterol is converted into pregnenolone in the adrenal glands, and then several enzymes complete the production of multiple hormones, including cortisol, aldosterone, estrogen, progesterone, and testosterone.

Assessing Your Thyroid Hormone Levels

Women between the ages of thirty and fifty are most likely to develop thyroid disorders, but they can occur in women both younger and older. Here is an overview of the particular thyroid measurements you want to include to assess your overall thyroid functioning:

Thyroid Stimulating Hormone (TSH) This is a thyroid hormone manufactured by the thyroid gland and indicates whether the thyroid is functioning normally.

Triiodothyronine (FT3) Active thyroid hormone T3 levels must remain within an optimal range in order to keep the body functioning properly; it is crucial to maintaining physical and mental health.

Free Thyroxine (FT4) Thyroxine is the main thyroid hormone produced by the thyroid. A well-regulated process causes thyroxine to generate the much more potent thyroid hormone T3.

Most women are treated with synthetic thyroid hormones, which is unfortunate, because there are natural thyroid supplements that can restore balance and function to the thyroid gland and its hormone production. Both DHEA and HGH supplements can also help restore thyroid levels and balance.

Assessing Melatonin Levels

Melatonin is typically tested through the saliva at three times during a twenty-four-hour period to reflect the natural rise and fall of melatonin with our circadian rhythm. Most of us are melatonin deficient, which can create sleep disturbances and other hormonal imbalances. The good news is that we can address this deficiency easily with supplementation. Typically, I advise my patients to begin with 1 mg of melatonin and see how it affects them. I tell my patients that they can ingest up to 10 mg of melatonin per night.

If you are taking too much melatonin, you might experience grogginess in the morning and nightmares during the night. Simply reduce the amount of melatonin. The side effects from melatonin can typically be relieved by adjusting dosage. Grogginess, mental sluggishness, sleepiness, and nightmares are the most common symptoms of too much melatonin. If you continue to suffer from sleep disturbances, consider asking your physician for DSIP, a peptide that helps the body restore its circadian rhythm.

A Quick Review of Hormonal Testing

BLOOD TESTS

Follicle-Stimulating Hormone (FSH)
Marker of perimenopause and menopause onset

Luteinizing Hormone (LH)
Marker of menopause onset

Sex Hormone–Binding Globulin (SHBG)
SHBG measures the overall amount of estrogen in your system. It is recommended that SHBG be tested along with testosterone in order to determine an imbalance between testosterone and estrogen.

Testosterone (Blood Spot) (T)
Testosterone levels can be assessed alone or in combination with SHBG to help determine imbalances of testosterone and estrogen.

Thyroid Hormones
Thyroid Stimulating Hormone (TSH)
Free Triiodothyronine (FT3)
Free Thyroxine (FT4)

Somatomedin C (IGF-1)
The IGF-1 test measures level of HGH.

SALIVA TESTS

Adrenal Stress Profile
In order to get the "big picture" of how your adrenal glands are functioning, I recommend combining a DHEA-S (DS) and cortisol in the morning (C1), noon (C2), evening (C3), and night (C4).

Diurnal Cortisol (Four Tests)
Cortisol is produced by the adrenal system and rises and falls throughout the day and night. By measuring cortisol in the morning (C1), noon (C2), evening (C3), and night (C4), this test can detect whether your experience of stress is chronic and pervasive.

AM/PM Cortisol
This cortisol test is a basic indicator of adrenal imbalance that tests cortisol in the morning (C1) and night (C4).

AM Cortisol (C)
This test is suggested for those suffering from situational stress and morning fatigue. It is a basic indicator of adrenal imbalance that tests cortisol in the morning (C1).

DHEA-S
Recommended with androgen deficiency or excess symptoms; indicator of stress level, mental performance, and insulin resistance.

Estradiol (E2)
The most predominant of the estrogens. Testing is recommended with symptoms of estrogen deficiency or excess and is best measured

along with progesterone, as an imbalance of these two hormones. Is associated with major symptoms of menopause and disorders of the reproductive system. Testing is also recommended when supplementing with a compounded preparation of bioidentical estrogens containing estradiol.

Estriol (E3)

It is recommended that estriol levels be measured when supplementing with a compounded preparation of bioidentical estrogens containing estriol.

Estrone (E1)

It is recommended that estrone levels be measured when supplementing with a compounded preparation of bioidentical estrogens.

Progesterone (Pg)

Recommended with symptoms of deficiency or excess. It's optimal to test progesterone along with estradiol, as an imbalance of these two hormones is associated with overall hormonal imbalance.

Testosterone (T)

Recommended with deficiency or excess symptoms, indicating low sex drive, hair loss/excess, muscle and bone status.

Hormone Levels and Dosage Recommendations

As I've mentioned, there is no "normal" or "typical" level or dosage for HRT. You need your own particular amount and combination of hormones, which may change over the course of a week, month, or year. The best way to understand whether you have sufficient amount of any one or combination of hormones is by monitoring your own symptoms and feelings. If your symptoms worsen or don't change at all, you should reach out to your practitioner. Especially in the first three to six months of HRT, it's optimal that you repeat certain tests and stay in close contact with your physician.

When patients begin working with me, it usually takes several months to refine their exact dosages. I depend on my patients to be conscientious in monitoring their symptoms and direct with me about what is going on with them physically, emotionally, and mentally. Their feedback is an important guide that helps me understand how to customize their treatment plan and keep them at optimal hormonal balance.

All women's treatments change over time. You may find that for a year or two certain dosages and combinations work well for you; then suddenly you notice new symptoms. That's when you return to your journal or log and to a quick scan of your records and reach out to your physician to report the changes. Your doctor will likely recommend getting your hormone levels checked and adjust your dosages according to what the tests reveal.

Problems with the Dosages of Chemicalized HRT

Over the past decade or so, physicians began to prescribe very low amounts of estrogen to diminish risks of breast cancer, cardiovascular disease, inflammation, weight gain, cognitive and memory problems, and other health hazards. But this low-dose regimen actually creates a "trap," a state of perpetual estrogen deficiency, which heightens a woman's risks for the very conditions she is seeking to avoid. As mentioned earlier, doctors came up with a so-called normal dosage of estrogen and progesterone based on a minority of patients. With a low dose of estrogen, you might well miss out on estrogen's benefits to cognitive health, mental and emotional balance, protection against disease, sexual invigoration, sound sleep, and youthful appearance—with youthful energy to match it.

Chemicalized estrogen is often delivered in a fixed dose, which does not match or respond to women's fluctuating estrogen needs. Especially during perimenopause and the early years of menopause, women's estrogen levels fluctuate frequently and often dramatically. The best way to manage this fluctuation is to deliver supplemental estrogen in a flexible dosing, which can change monthly and sometimes even weekly. Bioidentical estrogen allows us to do just this. I work closely with my patients to help them continually identify and update the dosing amounts—and mechanisms—that meet their individual hormonal needs.

Chemicalized estrogen in pill form leads to a sharp rise in SHBG, which binds up other important hormones (thyroid, testosterone, HGH), lowering their levels so they are unavailable to support health and hormone balance. And chemicalized estrogen in oral form may elevate blood pressure and increase risk for blood clots. Further, the estrogen patch can lead to skin rashes at the site. These patches often do not stay affixed to the skin and fall off before the dosing is done. Patches also deliver a fixed dose that may not provide enough estrogen to address symptoms.

Deciding on How You Want Your Hormones

You and your physician will decide which form of supplemental HRT will work best for you: oral supplements, skin patches, creams, or injections. These decisions will take into account your hormonal profile, the amount of hormone you need to overcome the deficiency, the optimal level you're aiming to maintain, the combination of hormones you need to take, and your personal preference. Some women don't mind injections;

others hate needles. Some women prefer oral supplements; others would rather apply a skin cream. Still others find creams messy and uncomfortable. I provide an overview of your options below.

TRANSDERMAL CREAMS

Transdermal creams are the most popular method for getting your hormone supplementation; however, you often don't absorb the first product you try. As a result, some women think it's not working. It's all about the absorption of a specific cream—no one cream works for everyone. Many of my patients—and I—prefer creams because they are directly absorbed through the skin and don't have to pass through the digestive system, which decreases their potency. Transdermal creams allow for more natural patterns of dosing. I recommend metered-dose pumps for the best accuracy and to make sure that the cream goes on smoothly so that it is absorbed quickly. It's best applied to the upper arm or inner forearm: rub the cream up and down on the arm until it's absorbed—typically in ten to twenty seconds.

While skin creams are easy to use, you have to careful not to let your partner, child, or pet come into contact with them as they can have adverse effects, especially estrogen and testosterone. Make sure children especially are shielded as they are already getting an unwanted xenoestrogen load from the environment that is harmful. Contact can occur skin to skin or from towels, clothing, or bedsheets and blankets. Just as men are cautioned not to let others in their household come into contact with their testosterone supplements, women have to guard against inadvertently transferring hormonal creams to others.

PATCHES

Patches have been quite popular with patients, because they are convenient and easy to use, and physicians also recommend them. However, some women find that over time they develop skin irritation from the patch, and the hormonal effects can be inconsistent, often delivering sub-optimal levels of hormone. Personally, I believe patches do not provide the same benefits for the mind, sleep cycle, and skin that other delivery options offer. I now avoid prescribing the patch because it tends to result in uneven hormone levels. Nonetheless, some of the brand names of bioidentical patch products include Alora, Climara, Esclim (generic), Estraderm, and Vivelle.

INJECTIONS

Injections of certain hormones, such as progesterone, are prescribed when appropriate for amenorrhea, uterine bleeding, and infertility treatment.

PILLS

Some physicians and women like the simplicity of pills for supplemental hormones, but I don't think they are effective at creating optimal levels of hormones. Because pills must pass through the digestive tract, the active part of the hormone is greatly diminished by the time it reaches the blood. The hormones in the pills are also hard on the liver, which breaks them down into metabolites, which may lead to other adverse effects. If you prefer pills for whatever reason, discuss with your physician the adjustments that you need to make in order for the pills to be both safe and effective.

PELLETS

Pellets are small, grain-size synthetic tablets that are implanted under the skin for three to six months at a time. Although some doctors believe that this method allows for consistent delivery, I worry because you can never know how well it's working—or not. I am also wary of its risks, which can include an association with cancer because of the accumulation of too high a level of hormones in the absence of estriol.

SUBLINGUAL DROPS AND LOZENGES

You can get your hormonal dose in a liquid form that you drop under your tongue, where the hormone is absorbed directly into the bloodstream. Achieving the proper dose is tricky since some drops are inevitably swallowed, and it's difficult to assess how much hormone gets absorbed. Another oral option is a lozenge, which you dissolve in your mouth, though it will take forty-five to sixty minutes to be fully absorbed. Some women prefer this method as they perceive it to be fast-acting, but it has the same disadvantage as drops do, in that you swallow some of the hormones, which then are lost in the digestive system.

TRANSMUCAL CREAMS

This cream is inserted vaginally through a suppository or as a topical cream inserted at the very opening of the vagina (first two inches). If the cream is inserted in the middle of the vagina, the substance is absorbed in the body, lessening its effect. Many fellow doctors and I believe vaginal creams are one of the best ways to treat overall menopause symptoms. It's a particularly effective way to dose progesterone, since it minimizes the side effect of drowsiness caused by this hormone. However, you do want to be considerate of your sexual partner and not use the suppository close to when you are going to be sexually active.

YOUR HEALTH JOURNAL: WHAT WORKS BEST FOR YOU

At this point in the book, you have assembled most of the basic information about your hormonal health, as well as the other conditions or medicines that you may be taking that can interact with your hormonal health. You are now ready to share this information with your health care provider or physician.

7

Building Your Body
with Food

I am neither a nutritionist nor a chef, but I am intensely committed to helping my patients—and you—get the best nutrition possible from the foods you eat. As I've mentioned, one of the most powerful ways to prevent disease, keep your estrogen and other hormones in balance, and fortify yourself against the effects of aging is through food. Healthy eating begins with making a commitment to yourself to build your body with food.

Let me be clear: I am not an absolutist. I love food and want to encourage you to love food, enjoy your meals, and savor a delicious variety of foods to delight your palate and your stomach. My approach offers you simple strategies to maintain your weight, lose pounds without deprivation or overthinking, or add calories to your diet if you can benefit from some healthy weight gain. Healthy eating ensures a healthy brain and body. You don't want to restrict types of food or get caught up in counting calories—typically those strategies backfire and only trigger obsessing about food. Building your body with food is also not about eating raw, going vegan, or drinking only green juice or fruit smoothies.

Healthy eating is about learning how a well-rounded selection of foods and satisfying meals will keep you healthy and also allow you to find the weight that is right for you. My approach is not a series of tricks to lose weight fast or a list of *eat this* and *don't eat that*. Whether you're a vegan, vegetarian, or carnivore, your eating strategy should incorporate a few fundamental principles: eat a diet that balances all food groups; moderate portion sizes; choose foods that are fresh, organic, and non-GMO, avoiding processed foods. When you stick to these three basic rules, you will end up making good choices. I'm going to ask you to emphasize lean proteins, such as fish, chicken, bison, and pork tenderloin—pasture-raised—and to limit dairy, sugar, starchy carbohydrates, and processed foods. I'm also going to introduce you to some important sources of good fats, such as olive oil, nuts, and seeds, which will help keep your blood sugar in balance, regulate your metabolism, and make your brain work better. The omega-3 fatty acids in these foods are protective against inflammation, cognitive decline, and hormonal imbalance. I also recommend that you increase your fiber intake to maintain proper digestion and improve your metabolism.

You will also find a guide to supplements—vitamins, minerals, and a probiotic—that will make up for anything missing in your diet and also reinforce a healthy gut, a crucial element to maintain hormonal balance, boost your ability to fight stress, and protect your overall health.

My approach to eating for wellness and hormonal balance works for women of all ages—whether you're in your twenties or forties or sixties. However, I have included some suggestions to keep in mind for each decade of health.

But my biggest message about food is this: it's meant to be enjoyed! I want you to embrace this approach to eating so that you can learn to love food again. Above all, you should think about food and eating as pleasurable! Many of my patients have been obsessed with fad diets, which usually restrict calories in order to lose unwanted pounds. I can say with great confidence that if you follow the general recommendations I have outlined, you will feel not only better (more balanced and without cravings) but also feel good, healthy, and fit.

The Perils of the Western Diet

Throughout this book, I've asked you to make a few key mind shifts, and one of the most important relates to how you think about food. Instead of thinking that you have to avoid certain foods, reduce the number of calories, and otherwise deprive yourself, think about food as a source of nutrition. And if we didn't live in a culture that is dominated by processed, packaged foods offered in jumbo sizes but, instead, ate a clean, plant-based diet of fresh foods, with just enough lean protein, good fats, and fiber, this mind shift would be easy. Unfortunately, we are up against a pervasive disease factory (yes, that's how I think of processed foods). The scientific evidence is clear: the typical "Western" diet, which is starchy and high in refined carbohydrates and sugar, relies heavily on red meat and processed meats, and includes "convenient" processed foods with chemical additives and unhealthful fats, is dangerous to health. The twin epidemics of obesity and type 2 diabetes clearly indicate the pervasive health hazards associated with the Western diet, which is typically consumed in big portions and strips even some healthful foods of their nutrient value through processing.

Keeping estrogen levels healthy is important for overall wellness and for brain health, but it will also help you eat a healthful diet. Estrogen influences levels of the hormone leptin, which is critical to appetite control. Leptin acts as a check against hunger, and it promotes feelings of fullness and satiety. When estrogen is deficient, leptin levels diminish—and hunger spikes. Low leptin triggers cravings for starchy, sugary, and fatty foods and a tendency to overeat and to binge eat. Low levels of leptin are also linked to an increased risk for neurodegeneration and neurodegenerative disease. At the same time, you don't want leptin levels to get too high. Chronically high leptin is associated with leptin resistance and obesity. When someone is severely overweight, the leptin-signaling mechanism breaks down. Even though there's plenty of leptin and plenty of stored fat (used for energy), your body gets triggered to eat.

Insulin resistance (IR) is another metabolic disorder that is related to hormone disruption. A common consequence of a high-sugar, high-carbohydrate diet, IR also destroys brain cells and impairs the brain's basic functioning. IR interferes with the brain's ability to consume glucose (glycogen), the fuel that powers the brain. IR also damages neurons that protect and facilitate memory. Both insulin resistance and diabetes are associated with cognitive impairment, memory problems, and neurodegeneration, including increased risk for Alzheimer's disease.

Excessive intake of refined carbohydrates (nonvegetable carbs) in processed foods is associated with health risks and chronic illness. A typical Western diet elevates a woman's risk for breast cancer, particularly for hormone-receptor-positive breast cancer.

In addition, a diet high in refined carbohydrates and sugars damages brain cells and brain function. Trans fats and saturated fats found in processed foods undermine memory and cognitive abilities. Red meat and dairy eaten frequently can cause similar damage. The typical Western diet is deficient in omega-3 fatty acids, which are found in fish, nuts, and healthy oils, and this deficiency is linked to cognitive decline. A diet high in saturated fat and sugar also lowers levels of BDNF (brain-derived neurotrophic factor), a protein that's essential to brain health and to the survival of neurons. BDNF actually worsens the effects of traumatic brain injury.

Women with type 2 diabetes are more likely to have problems with brain function and memory. Indeed, studies show that women with diabetes and metabolic syndrome show more frequent signs of early cognitive decline. But people with type 2 diabetes perform better cognitively after consuming a single, low-glycemic, low-carbohydrate meal.

The classic Western diet, which is made up of more than 50 percent starchy or sweet, nonfibrous carbs, is at the root of a host of illnesses:

- Insulin resistance
- Metabolic syndrome
- Diabetes
- Inflammation
- Arthritis
- High cholesterol
- High blood pressure
- High blood sugar
- Colon cancer
- Cognitive degeneration
- Chronic overweight and obesity

Excess carbohydrate consumption, even in early life, can increase a child's vulnerability to obesity and insulin resistance throughout her adult life.

In contrast, my approach to eating, which is a blend of Mediterranean and keto diets, has many benefits for your health. When you emphasize lots of organic vegetables, eat just enough lean protein, include sufficient good fats, and reduce sugar and starchy carbs, you will

- Support, protect, and enhance your cognitive function
- Lift your mood
- Manage your stress more effectively
- Protect yourself against cancer
- Reduce your risk for cardiovascular disease
- Lose weight or maintain a healthy weight
- Improve your overall quality of life

Signs That Weight Gain and Dietary Challenges Are Hormone Related

Estrogen and other hormone imbalances can lead to weight gain at many points throughout a woman's life. Here are some indications of when weight gain is likely to be tied to your hormones:

- Weight gain of five pounds or more in the week before menstruation
- Strong cravings for sweets, starches, or savory carbohydrates in the week before a period
- Weight gain during perimenopause and menopause
- Weight gain of more than five pounds while taking oral contraceptives

Mediterranean Meets Keto

I like to think of my approach to healthy eating as "Mediterranean meets keto." For years, my family and I have followed a Mediterranean diet that is rich in healthy omega-3 fats from olive oil and nuts and emphasizes seasonal, simple dishes that are easy to make from local produce and that include fish, poultry, and lean meats. This way of eating has also worked well for most of my patients. However, in the past few years, I've updated my approach because I've found that many of my patients need more direction in creating meals that rely on these basic dietary building blocks. Whereas the Mediterranean diet allows for moderate amounts of grains and legumes (pasta, lentils, chickpeas, and other beans), keto takes a narrower stance, reducing or eliminating these altogether. A ketogenic diet is a very low-carb diet designed to put your body in fat-burning mode. When you take out sugar and starchy carbohydrates from pasta and bread, for instance, your body has less glucose to rely on for energy. In this low-glucose state, it will signal the liver to produce ketones, energy molecules that metabolize fat. (If you have type 1 diabetes, take medicine for high blood pressure, or are breast-feeding, do not do a keto diet.)

Although I believe either of these two approaches is healthy and will support your hormonal balance, you need to discover for yourself which one actually makes you feel better. Gloria, a thirty-eight-year-old patient of mine, has metabolic syndrome (a group of conditions that are tied to insulin resistance); years of being overweight and sedentary led to this cluster of symptoms, which makes it difficult for her to process starchy carbs and sugar. So for her a strict keto approach works best. Ariel, who is forty-six, has always been active and her weight is steady. She can enjoy pasta once or even twice a week and an occasional sweet dessert without feeling sluggish or putting on weight. The Mediterranean approach, which allows for more sugar and carbs, works great for her. In contrast, if Gloria eats even a small portion of pasta, she feels "puffy" the next day and begins to crave bread.

You might be like Gloria or like Ariel or somewhere in between. As you take on the mind-set that food is nutrition—enjoyable nutrition—pay attention to how your eating different foods makes you feel. Keep notes in your journal. Write down your responses to a meal: Did you feel sated or satisfied? Were you hungry an hour later? Did you feel sluggish or bloated the day after? Are you experiencing any food cravings?

And while I don't want you to go "scale crazy," weighing yourself can be helpful to see how certain foods agree with you or not. Keep a record of where you are when you start this healthy eating approach and how you fare over the next six months. You might make special note of where you are in your cycle when you have any reactions to certain foods or, if you are menopausal, how these reactions change as you start your HRT and make any adjustments to it with your doctor.

Without a doubt, low estrogen and other hormone deficiencies make it more difficult for women to lose weight, and they make it all too easy to gain weight. Estrogen deficiency triggers other changes in hormones that alter appetite and can make you feel more inclined to eat the "wrong" foods and to eat too much of them. Unhealthful eating and excess weight are catalysts for other health issues—high blood pressure, metabolic problems, and insulin resistance among them—and also may wear down your confidence, energy, pride in your body and appearance, interest in physical exercise, and desire for sex.

As a culture, we need to enhance our awareness of the power of vegetables as a rich source of nutrients and fiber. The cheapest food we can buy is vegetables—and there is so much natural variability in their colors, smells, and taste for us to enjoy.

Bioidentical Hormones Suppress Appetite

Research demonstrates that bioidentical estrogen has a direct effect on appetite control, influencing the hormones that govern hunger and satiety—without incurring the unwanted, unhealthful side effects that come with chemicalized estrogens.

Applied directly to the skin in gel or cream, bioidentical estrogen lowers ghrelin levels, reducing hunger and cravings. Ghrelin is a fast-acting hormone that stimulates hunger. Bioidentical estrogen can lower food intake, and it increases levels of CCK (cholecystokinin), a protein that helps digest fats and proteins and promotes satiety.

The diet–estrogen connection works in both directions. Not only do estrogen levels affect diet, the choices you make about what foods to eat and drink influence estrogen. A poor, unbalanced diet can undermine estrogen and other hormone balance to the detriment of your health. Eating unhealthful foods, including processed foods, introduces estrogen-mimicking chemicals and environmental estrogens into the body. And, as you've seen, these so-called foreign invaders also mess up your hormonal balance.

What Does Mediterranean + Keto Look Like?

The foundations of the Mediterranean + keto diet are whole, unprocessed foods that do not come preprepared, wrapped in plastics, or sealed in boxes. These foods aren't made in factories. They are grown in fields and groves or harvested from the ocean. They are in-season juicy fruits and plump vegetables, hearty legumes, rich nuts, green-golden oils, and whole, unprocessed grains. A Mediterranean + keto diet does include animal proteins—primarily fish but also organic, free-range poultry and pasture-raised beef and bison, as well as organic eggs. Your good fats from omega-3 fatty acids come in olives and olive oils, nuts and seeds, and certain fruits, like avocados and coconut. Dairy is not a heavy-duty staple of either approach, but enjoying a piece of hard cheese every now and then is not off-limits.

Starchy vegetables (potatoes, corn, and squash, for example), sweets, and alcohol are consumed only in moderation, if at all. The Mediterranean diet avoids processed foods and their refined and processed sugars, saturated fats and oils, and the chemical additives that are associated with serious and chronic health problems. Keto is further restrictive since it does not include any grains, sweets, or alcohol.

Hundreds of studies over the years have demonstrated the health benefits of the Mediterranean diet, including a reduction in the incidence of diabetes, cardiovascular disease, and some cancers (colon and intestinal, for example). Scientists have also shown that a Mediterranean diet slows aging and can significantly increase longevity.

The Mediterranean diet is also enjoyable, which is just as important. The foods and eating habits allow you to savor and delight in food while also eating mindfully, moderately, and healthfully. Eating the Mediterranean way means creating meals from simple, whole ingredients and then sitting down—ideally with human company and without electronic and digital distractions—to take the time to enjoy the food and connections to other people. Feeling good about food and about the rituals of eating can make a significant difference in how you feel and how you eat. Principles like moderation, portion control, and the discipline to say no to favorite indulgences—all key to weight management and good dietary habits—are a great deal easier to execute when you do them as part of a larger experience of enjoyment and pleasure.

You don't need to reside on a Tuscan hillside or a pastoral Greek village to enjoy these foods and way of eating. Local, seasonal, and organic fruits and vegetables are available at farmers' markets and at grocery stores, since the large-scale food purveyors have recognized the demand for organic produce and meats and for foods grown close to home. For a Mediterranean diet, you stock simple, easy-to-procure foods in your pantry: beans and other legumes, high-quality olive oil and other oils, nuts, herbs and spices.

Whether you live in a big-city high-rise or a multigenerational family home along a suburban street, you need to make only one basic commitment: to slow down long enough to taste and savor the food you're eating, to relax with family or friends—or your own good company—and to take pleasure in feeding yourself well.

The Benefits of Keto

Recent studies have supported the health benefits of a keto diet low in starchy carbs, high in protein and fat, and high in fiber from vegetables; studies have shown

- Weight maintenance or loss, if desired
- Reversal of type 2 diabetes
- Lowering of blood pressure
- Management of epilepsy
- Reversal of polycystic ovary syndrome
- Reduction of irritable bowel syndrome
- Improvement to acne

The 30-30-30 Rule

Let's take a closer look at the makeup of the Mediterranean + keto approach. Essentially, I recommend a roughly even split among the major dietary components:

30 percent protein

30 percent fat

30 percent fiber in the form of fiber-rich vegetables and/or
  whole grains

The remaining 10 percent? That's where a little flexibility comes into play. That 10 percent makes room for a glass of wine with dinner, an occasional dessert, a once-in-a-while side of mashed potatoes or bowl of pasta. None of us will eat perfectly every meal of every day. Better to leave a little room for small deviations from your daily eating than to be so strict you abandon healthful practices altogether. Make a real commitment to eating the right foods, in moderate amounts, and do the best you can to live out that commitment at each meal, knowing you have a little flexibility to keep you on track.

Your first 30 percent building block is protein. *Protein* should primarily come from wild-caught fish and lean, organic pork and chicken. The occasional indulgence in red meat should also come from an organic or grass-finished source. (Grass-fed often means the animals were grain fed for most of their lives and then given grass just before being slaughtered.) Animals raised to provide organic meat are raised in open pastures, where their diet comes from grass—not grain or corn. They are free of antibiotics and genetically modified components. Their food is grown without use of chemical pesticides and fertilizers. These products cost more, but they are an important investment in your health. Eggs, especially egg whites, can also provide your diet with protein. Dairy is a source of protein best used in moderation, as is soy. Although soy has been described as having links to cancer, it's my opinion that these associations are misleading. Soy is a wonderful source of vegetarian protein, though I do recommend you rely on organic, non-GMO sources. Indeed, I suspect that any cancer links from soy are not related to soy as much as they are to the chemicals that accompany nonorganic, pesticide-riddled sources.

Fat is an essential part of your diet, both for health and satisfaction. Fat protects and fuels the brain, helps the body absorb other nutrients, protects the integrity of your body's cells, and provides a potent source of energy. Chefs say that "fat is flavor." They're right. The key is to use healthy, hormone-supporting fat sources. For these, look first and foremost to the Mediterranean diet and its olives and olive oil, nuts, and seeds (like flax and chia), and coconut and avocados. The wild-caught fish and lean animal proteins you'll be eating provide additional sources of healthy fats. Organic coconut and coconut oil are having a renaissance, and you can find oils to cook with, blend into a smoothie, or use as part of a salad dressing. And even though I don't want you to do a lot of snacking, a handful of nuts—almonds, cashews, macadamia—is a great source of healthful dietary fat and protein.

The 30 percent of your diet that is *fibrous* **carbohydrates** should come primarily from organic vegetable sources rather than grains. Vegetables supply the broad base of nutrients your body needs each day as well as complex carbohydrates that fill the body with fiber and deliver a steady source of energy. The importance of fiber to your diet is hard to overstate. Fiber supports cardiovascular health, aids in healthy digestion and elimination, controls blood sugar, and can lower the risks for some cancers. High-fiber vegetables are low in calories, but their fiber content contributes to a feeling of fullness after eating, which can help you avoid the cravings and perpetual hunger that come from consuming simple carbohydrates in processed grains and sugar.

Dark leafy greens, cruciferous vegetables such as broccoli and cauliflower, vine-ripened tomatoes, hearty root vegetables such as carrots, turnips, and sweet potato—these you can eat richly, abundantly, and with satisfying variety while on a plant-based diet.

Also, consider replacing potatoes and rice with fibrous veggies such as celery root, rutabaga, and parsnips—these vegetables offer wonderful flavor and texture without the high glycemic effect on your blood sugar.

You'll see plenty of soups among my meal suggestions, because they are a convenient, satisfying way to pack vegetables into your daily eating plan.

Organic fruit is actually a carbohydrate, but it does have a place in your diet. It's important to manage fruit intake carefully, because the body treats fruit just as it does the sugar in alcohol, in terms of how it is broken down and processed. That's an indication of how you should incorporate fruit into your dietary routine: give it the limited space you give to alcohol, whether you have a glass of wine or a piece of fruit as dessert.

It is not necessary to eliminate all grain-based carbohydrates, including wheat, from your diet (unless you have a gluten sensitivity or celiac disease, which you should address with your physician). Wheat and other grains should comprise a small share of your overall carbohydrate intake. When you do eat grains, opt for organic whole grains rather than processed grain products. You're better off eating brown rice, toasted barley, or steel-cut oats than sandwich bread or store-bought pasta. I encourage you to branch out beyond wheat products to try other grains, including farro, amaranth, and different varieties of wild rice. These whole grains are satisfying, satiating, and fiber-rich and can add welcome variety to your diet while limiting the amount of gluten you consume.

As I mention above, the remaining 10 percent of your meal is up to you. I recommend that on some days or evenings you give yourself a treat—whether that's pasta, a glass of wine, or dessert. On other nights, up your veggies and skip that starchy carb altogether. You are going to be able to trust yourself as you become tuned in to how certain foods make you feel.

On Eating Fish

One of the most important elements of a Mediterranean diet is eating as much fish as possible; it's a great source of lean protein, omega-3 fatty acids, and other nutrients. These potent sources of omega-3 fatty acids offer powerful protection against disease, help the brain maintain its full function, and protect physiological health at the cellular level. I recommend eating fish at least once a week. There are a few important considerations to keep in mind when purchasing fish.

Buy wild-caught. These fish carry far greater amounts of healthy fish oil and omega-3 fats than farmed fish do. Farmed fish also have a higher concentration of unhealthful omega-6 fats than their wild counterparts. Farmed fish are fed antibiotics and, over their life span, accumulate significantly higher levels of toxins and pollutants through the water than wild fish do. Farming fish such as salmon creates a great demand for smaller wild fish to feed the farmed fish. This has led to overfishing of feeder fish such as sardines, mackerel, and others, damaging ecosystems and undermining wild fish populations as a whole. Keep in mind that there is no such thing as "Atlantic Salmon"—salmon do not live in the Atlantic Ocean. Fish marketed this way are typically chemicalized fish.

Pick fish low on the food chain. Smaller fish typically fall lower on the food chain than larger fish do. Small fish are less contaminated by mercury and other toxins. Anchovies, sardines, and shrimp are some good examples of smaller fish that are potent sources of nutrition.

Choose sustainable seafood. Supporting sustainable fisheries is one way to protect the health of the oceans and their fish populations. Standing at the fish counter and trying to determine what is the most sustainable choice can be daunting. There are resources that can simplify the process.

Four Rules for Healthy Weight

Any approach to eating well should be simple. These four rules can be your guide to making healthy choices that help you either lose or maintain weight.

Eat meals. Although some new diets recommend eating five meals a day, including two snacks, our bodies are not really designed to take in and digest food so frequently. Digestion takes a lot of energy and time. The key is to eat whole meals that are satisfying so that you don't really need to eat snacks. The only people who should snack are those who are prone to severe hypoglycemia. Ideally, there should be about twelve hours between breakfast and dinner. Snacking makes it more difficult to keep an accurate assessment of what you're eating during the day and raises overall daily calorie consumption. Snacking contributes to weight gain and makes it harder to lose weight and keep weight off. Snacking may also reinforce tendencies to eat under emotional stress. Instead of relying on snacks to keep you satisfied, focus on high-fiber meals that don't skimp on healthy fats. Keep in mind that most extra pounds come from overconsumption of protein and non-fibrous (aka starchy) carbohydrates, so, as you will see in my meal plan, I have emphasized vegetables and healthy fats, avoiding too much protein and/or carbs. If you want to lose weight by resetting your body's natural satiety signals, you may want to investigate a simple version of intermittent fasting, in which you skip breakfast and eat two simple meals a day.

Stay hydrated. You need to drink plenty of water. A general rule of thumb is five eight-ounce glasses of water per day. Water detoxifies your body's organs—from your skin to your liver. Water helps keep your digestion engine and metabolism moving. It also helps fight against the environmental pollutants that advance aging. However, many of my patients have trouble accomplishing this feat. I point out that water is contained in a lot of their vegetables and fruit and other water-dense foods. What's key is learning to stay properly hydrated. There's a new fad to drink alkaline or electrolyte water; helping your body balance an acidic environment with this type of water is a good idea, but you never want to drink this water with a meal, as you need an acidic environment to digest your food properly. A great way to set up your digestion for the day is to drink room-temperature water with some lemon or vinegar; this primes your digestive system and aids metabolism. You can also enjoy the health benefits of coffee and tea. In particular, green tea and coffee contain ingredients that have been shown to have anti-inflammatory, anticancer, and anticholesterol properties.

Learn to say no to sugar. Food can be described as either high-glycemic or low-glycemic, according to how strongly it signals your body to convert sugar into glucose. If a food produces a strong and immediate insulin response, it is considered high-glycemic; if a food contains fiber, protein, or fat, it will have a low-glycemic effect on your body. My approach to eating is low-glycemic because it encourages you to avoid starchy and sweet foods that have a strong insulin response and then flood your body with excess glucose. When blood sugar gets too high, not only do you experience cravings for more sugar but also your body becomes somewhat addicted to the "high" of blood sugar. Chronic high blood sugar is truly alarming in its capacity to cause damage to the body. Regular and excessive consumption of sugar—particularly refined sugars—taxes the metabolic and cardiovascular systems, suppresses immune function, and contributes to inflammation. Sugar consumption accelerates aging and is a contributor to most diseases.

If you have trouble saying no to sugar, you are not alone. However, the more you consume fresh vegetables, lean protein, and healthy fats, the less you will crave sugar. You will also keep your blood sugar in balance and avoid the inflammatory states that cause the illnesses listed here. Women may be especially vulnerable to sugar addiction because of cravings that occur as a result of fluctuating hormones during menstruation, pregnancy, perimenopause, and menopause.

Choose your meats wisely. I enjoy steak. That's the simple truth. I would love to tuck into a hearty T-bone on a regular basis, but I do it only occasionally. Red meat is higher in calories and in saturated fats than other leaner animal proteins. It is also particularly unhealthful when consumed regularly, in part because of its nutritional content and in part because of the manner in which it is often cooked. Recently, the World Health Organization classified processed or non-grass-finished meat—including beef, pork, and lamb—as a likely carcinogen, and a probable cause of colorectal cancer. In the same step, the WHO classified processed meats—meats that have been cured or otherwise processed into products such as bacon, sausage, and hot dogs—as definite carcinogens that contribute significantly to colorectal cancer risk. Eating meat regularly (more than three times per week) raises risk for breast cancer dramatically: eating 1.5 servings of red meat daily elevates breast cancer risk by 97 percent. Regular red meat consumption also increases cardiovascular disease, elevates risk for diabetes, and is associated with shorter life span than vegetarian diets.

Does this mean all meat should come off the table? No, but if you're a regular meat eater, it's time to switch to grass-finished sources, replace meat with wild-caught fish, or try plant-based protein sources, such as high-protein grains like quinoa, wheatberry, and farro, or legumes, such as lentils and chickpeas.

Good nutrition is the foundation of health. Many people would avoid many chronic diseases such as diabetes, heart disease, and cancers such as breast cancer and colon cancer by reducing their consumption of meat (especially processed meat) and increasing their consumption of fresh vegetables and fruits. Most of all, we need to relearn to enjoy this way of eating!

Your Shopping List

The Mediterranean + keto way of eating includes a tremendous variety of foods. It's a diet full of different colors, textures, and tastes. Here is a shopping list to guide you and prep you for the meal plans below.

When choosing your protein sources, try to purchase grass-finished or certified organic meats, including beef, poultry, and pork. When selecting fish, try to obtain wild-caught, with an emphasis on smaller fish less contaminated by mercury and other toxins. In shopping for vegetables, choose organic and in-season vegetables whenever possible, including dark and leafy green vegetables, root vegetables (squash, turnip, carrots), celery and celeriac, tomatoes, eggplant, onions, peppers, and garlic.

Your herbs should be local or organic, fresh or dried, including cilantro, parsley, basil, thyme, rosemary, dill, mint, tarragon, and others, used regularly and in abundance to season food and reduce reliance on fat, sugar, and salt for flavor.

Legumes come in many varieties. They too should be organic or non-GMO, such as lentils, black-eyed peas, black beans, chickpeas, kidney beans, and others, preferably dried, not canned or pre-cooked, unless the label states that the packaging is nonharmful.

Nuts and seeds, including flaxseed, walnuts, almonds, hazel-nuts, and others, preferably raw and unsalted, should also be lo-cally sourced, organic, and non-GMO. This is true of your other fat sources, too, including olive oil, olives, grape-seed oil, and co-conut and coconut oil. Chia seeds should also be organic.

Here's your list!

30% Protein List
Animal Proteins (Protein + Fat)
Beef
Bison
Buffalo
Chicken
Eggs
Pork
Turkey

Legumes (Protein + Fat + Fiber)
Adzuki beans
Black beans
Cannellini (white) beans
Chickpeas (garbanzo)
Kidney beans
Lentils
Lima beans
Navy beans
Pinto beans

30 Percent Fiber-Rich Carb List

Nonstarchy Vegetables (Carb + Fiber + Protein)

Artichokes

Arugula

Asparagus

Bamboo shoots

Bean sprouts

Beet greens

Bell peppers (red, yellow, green)

Broccoli

Brussels sprouts

Cabbage

Carrots

Cauliflower

Celery

Collard greens

Cucumber

Eggplant

Endive

Fennel

Flaxseed

Green beans

Kale

Leeks

Lettuce

Mushrooms

Mustard greens

Onions

Radicchio

Radishes

Shallots

Spaghetti squash
Spinach
Squash (acorn, butternut, winter)
Summer squash
Swiss chard
Tomatoes
Turnips
Turnip greens
Watercress
Zucchini

30 Percent Fat List
Fats (Fat + Carb + Fiber) to Enjoy at Each Meal
Avocado
Avocado oil
Chia seed
Coconut oil
Cultured or pastured organic butter
Flaxseed oil
Freshly ground flaxseed meal
Ghee (clarified butter)
MCT oil (highly refined, nutrient-dense coconut oil)
Olive oil (extra-virgin if used in salads)
Olives
Raw nuts: bulk raw almonds, cashews, pecans, walnuts,
    macadamia, Brazil nuts, pistachios

**High-fiber, Starchy Carbohydrate Choices to Enjoy in Moderation
(1–2 times per week)**
Gluten-free pasta
Sweet potatoes, yams

Your 10 Percent List

Low-Fiber Starchy Carbohydrates to Enjoy in Limited Quantities

Bread

California basmati rice, California wild rice, or sushi rice

Corn

Pasta

White potatoes

Fruits (Enjoy in Moderation)

Apples

Bananas

Blackberries

Blueberries

Boysenberries

Cherries

Grapes

Lemon

Lime

Nectarines

Oranges

Peaches

Pears

Pineapples

Plums

Pomegranates

Raspberries

Strawberries

Tangerines

Watermelon

Supplements For Your Brain

Recently, scientists have been focusing on certain supplements that prevent the aging of the brain. In particular, these supplements have been shown to improve memory and neurogenesis (the creation of new neurons). Take as directed.

Acetyl-L-Carnitine and Huperzine A (acetylcholine)

Aniracetam

Centrophenoxine

Cerebrolysine (peptide)

Dihexa (or Angiotensin IV peptide)

Galantamine

Ginkgo biloba

HVMN (peptide)

Magnesium

Taurine

Transresveratrol

Semax (peptide)

Sulforaphane

Vinpocetine

Vitamin D

Your Guide to Supplements

Ideally, we would get all our nutrients from the foods we eat daily and not need to supplement with vitamins and minerals. But for the vast majority of us—even those of us who are committed to eating healthfully and avoiding foods that can cause us harm—a diet that delivers all the necessary nutrients in abundance just isn't realistically obtainable. We are faced with continual, increasing depletion of nutrients from soil due to pollutants, chemicals, and toxins, which leads to nutrient-deficient or even toxic foods. Toxins in fresh water and the oceans also affect the quality of nutrition we can obtain from wild or farmed foods. For instance, children and pregnant women should not eat freshwater fish because of the high occurrence of mercury in those fish, and certain large-finned ocean fish are also contaminated with mercury. So our bodies need reinforcements, more protective power, to successfully thwart these toxic threats to health. The dosages provided are in line with the amounts that I most often suggest for my patients, but your individual requirements may be different, so always consult with your health care provider about your specific needs.

B complex Supports adrenal health, assists the body in converting food to energy, improves and protects cognitive function, lowers a woman's risk for breast cancer.

In food: egg whites, lean meats (including poultry), fish, cabbage, lentils, soybeans

Supplement: 25–100 mg daily with food

A full B complex includes B5, B6, B12, and a methylated form of folic acid.

Coenzyme Q10 CoQ10 is a powerful antioxidant and a critical nutrient for cellular health. Studies show CoQ10 protects against breast cancer and extends the survival time for women with breast cancer. People who take statins, beta-blockers, and antidepressant medications have diminished levels of this important enzyme and should often supplement.

Supplement: 100–300 mg daily with food

Turmeric Turmeric, the vibrant orange spice used in Indian and other Southeast Asian cuisines, is a potent anti-inflammatory. It has been shown to improve memory, cognitive function, and learning capacity and protect the nervous system from oxidative stress. Turmeric slows and prevents bone loss. It protects against diabetes, lowers triglyceride levels, and reduces cholesterol. Turmeric boosts levels of vitamins C and E and helps prevent cancer. This nutrient slows aging at the cellular level and extends life span.

Supplement: 600 mg daily with food

Vitamin C This antioxidant protects against breast cancer and lowers breast cancer mortality. It contributes to vascular and cardiovascular health and protects healthy brain function.

In food: dark and leafy greens, citrus fruits, berries, kiwifruit, broccoli, tomatoes

Supplement: 1,000 mg daily

Vitamin D An anti-inflammatory, vitamin D helps protect against breast cancer, skin cancer, and prostate cancer. Vitamin D slows the growth of breast cancers and other cancers. This vitamin offers protection against autoimmune disease and slows aging. Vitamin D is highly protective to the brain, helping dispose of beta-amyloid protein and protecting myelin levels in the brain. It also protects against bone loss and improves muscle strength and mood. Test for vitamin D levels before starting a supplement routine in order to identify the correct dosage. The optimal range is 60–80 ng/mL, and women should not exceed 100 ng/mL. If you are taking more than 1,000 iu daily, do so only in consultation with a physician. And always pair vitamin D with vitamin K or you risk building up calcium deposits in places you don't want, including the blood vessels!

DHA/EPA (Fish Oil) Anti-inflammatory, with broad and powerful health benefits and protections to cardiovascular health and cognitive health and function. Also has been shown to reduce risks for breast cancer and slow breast cancer growth.

Supplement: 1,000–2,000 mL daily

Ginkgo Biloba Provides cancer protection, including against colon and ovarian cancers. Increases oxygen supply to the brain, works to protect and improve memory and to slow age-related memory loss. Increases antioxidants and reduces oxidative stress and inflammation throughout the body, including the brain. May help treat migraine. Follow the suggested amount on the product.

Vitamin K Helps build bone and can treat osteoporosis. Provides protection to brain health. Offers cancer protection and protects cardiovascular health. Improves insulin sensitivity.

In food: leafy green vegetables, cruciferous vegetables, tomatoes, turnips, parsley (raw), vegetable oils, including olive, soybean, canola, and cottonseed. Hydrogenated oils decrease the body's ability to absorb vitamin K.

Supplement: 75–150 mcg daily with food

Magnesium Magnesium is a powerful enhancer to overall physiological function. This mineral reduces stress, improves sleep, helps the body absorb nutrients, and moves the bowels for better removal of waste.

In food: legumes, dark leafy greens, fish, nuts. Also found in whole grains and oats.

Supplement: 400–1,000 mg daily with food. Start with the lowest dose and work gradually upward if necessary. Signs that magnesium dose is too high are diarrhea, very soft stool, unusual sleepiness in the daytime or at times when one would expect to be alert.

Quercetin This bioflavonoid provides protection against breast and other cancers and may treat cancers. Working to boost the effectiveness of resveratrol, quercetin also can help minimize the damage to the body from oxidative stress. Quercetin reduces inflammation, protects against neurodegeneration, and reduces hypertension. Follow the dosage suggestion on the product packaging.

Transresveratrol This antioxidant is found in the skins of grapes and other berries and is considered part of the explanation for the "French paradox"—the combination of low cardiovascular disease combined with a diet high in saturated fat that exists in France. Transresveratrol protects brain function and health and lowers inflammation throughout the body, and specifically in the brain after injury. Transresveratrol protects against breast cancer and encourages apoptosis, or healthy cell death. This compound can help improve sleep and strengthen sleep-wake cycles. It also may reduce polycystic ovary syndrome.

Supplement: up to 50 mg daily with food

Tocotrienol E and Vitamin E Complex An antioxidant, vitamin E helps prevent cancer and slows cancer growth. This combination provides a complete range of necessary vitamin E compounds, including gamma, delta, and alpha E. Vitamin E functions as a strong antioxidant and promotes brain health.

In food: nuts and seeds and their oils, including sunflower seeds and almonds and their oils; spinach; beet greens; collard greens; fish; wheat germ; olive oil

Supplement: 400–800 iu E complex and 100 mg tocotrienol E daily with food.

Supplements for Weight Loss and Weight Management

These supplements can further boost your metabolism and help you burn calories, improving weight loss. For all supplements, follow the directions on the product for dosage.

Curcumin: decreases body fat, lowers risk for obesity

Transresveratrol: helps optimize metabolic function

ALA (alpha lipoic acid): spurs weight loss, increases insulin sensitivity

L-arginine: decreases body fat

Lovida

Eating Right Throughout Your Life

The Mediterranean + keto approach is optimal, no matter how old you are or what kinds of hormone supplements you begin. Its holistic, nutrient-rich combinations support long-term hormonal balance, achievement of a healthy weight, and resistance to illness and disease. That said, there are nutritional and dietary priorities that change with age and hormonal life stages. Below are the modifications that are relevant to you now and into the future.

Your Twenties and Thirties: The Childbearing Years

This is the time to create a strong foundation of dietary health and balanced eating habits. In your twenties, metabolism is as robust as it will ever be in your adult lifetime, but don't let that lead you astray from healthful eating. Rather than use this time to indulge in processed foods loaded with sugar and additives, use your young adulthood to establish the eating practices you'll rely on for the rest of your life. Learn to cook, invest in organic foods, and keep your sugar indulgence to a minimum.

During these years, you should pay particular attention to eating a diet that includes the following nutrients:

Calcium: Food sources include eggs, tofu, almonds, salmon, cabbage, yogurt, milk

Iron: Food sources include dark greens, whole grains, oats, and lean protein in fish, chicken, and pork

Folate: Food sources include dark greens, citrus, tomatoes, legumes, whole grains

Vitamin C: Food sources include peppers, citrus, tomato

Your Forties: Perimenopause

During your forties, it becomes increasingly important to maintain a healthy weight. It also becomes more difficult, thanks to a slowing metabolism and wildly fluctuating hormones. During this decade, you should focus on the following:

Avoiding sugar. This will help keep inflammation in check, reduce uncontrolled appetite and cravings that lead to weight gain, and diminish fatigue and energy crashes.

Limiting starchy carbs and salt. Processed and high-starch grains contribute to bloating, which is common for women in their forties and women in perimenopause. Steer clear of processed grains like pasta and bread or any grain that causes you to bloat. Salty foods also make bloating worse.

No snacking. Planning healthful, satisfying meals will help you feel satisfied and less likely to need to snack throughout the day, which can easily lead to weight gain.

Your Fifties, Sixties, and Beyond: Menopause

During these years, pay particular attention to eating for brain health and bone health. With metabolism continuing to slow, portion control becomes especially important to keeping weight in check.

Avoid foods that trigger menopause symptoms. Certain foods, including alcohol, chocolate, caffeine, and some spicy foods, can exacerbate night sweats and hot flashes.

Up your healthy fats and fiber. These dietary components will help you feel full and satiated, while also promoting healthy digestion.

Support your bones. Consuming foods rich in calcium, magnesium, vitamin D, and vitamin K can help protect bone strength with age. Wild-caught fish, organic soy foods, nuts and seeds, and dark greens are among the best sources of these minerals and vitamins when you are in your fifties and sixties. Limit caffeine and alcohol to limit bone loss and to avoid blocking absorption of nutrients like calcium that support bones.

Eat for your brain. Many of the foods that support bone health also provide protection for the brain. Focus on lean proteins and healthy fats, from wild-caught fish, organic animal proteins, and organic soy products. Omega-3 fats and fatty acids are essential for brain health. In addition to wild-caught fish, avocados, nuts, and seeds are excellent sources of omega-3s.

Consume organic phytoestrogens. Food sources of estrogen can help supplement the dwindling estrogen in your body. Organic soy products are a good source of phytoestrogens, as are many seeds, including pumpkin, sesame, and sunflower.

YOUR HEALTH JOURNAL: MINDFUL EATING

I highly recommend using your journal as a place to record the foods you eat. Especially as you begin your shift into healthy eating—whether or not you follow my Mediterranean + keto plan to the letter or not—making a habit of thinking about your food choices can have a positive impact on feeling more in control of how you eat, when you eat, and how much you eat. Soon, you may not need such attention to detail. However, any change in habit and the formation of a new habit takes conscious effort and a willingness to be aware.

8

A Four-Week Meal Plan

Tʜɪs meal plan combines foods that complement both a Mediterranean, whole foods approach and a streamlined keto approach that emphasizes lean protein and good fats. Again, Mediterranean allows for grains, legumes, and other starchy carbs in moderation, whereas a strict keto approach includes no grains at all. Both approaches include fiber in the form of vegetables and some fruits. I've tried to offer you variety while also keeping the meal suggestions simple and efficient so that you can keep your trips to the grocery store to a minimum.

You will note that some dishes are marked with an asterisk (*); these are accompanied by recipes in the Resources section at the back of the book. I've made these recipes easy to prepare in less than twenty minutes. Other dishes are marked by two asterisks (**); these items refer to good store-bought brands that I trust because they are organic, contain no genetically modified additives, and are minimally processed. A list of these brand-name products can also be found in Resources.

Whenever possible, I have included leftovers to cut down on the need for meal preparation; in such cases, I've included enough servings in the recipe. (Recipes are always adjustable for serving size.)

Feel free to add any herbs, including ground or coarse black pepper, for taste. Use sea salt sparingly (a little pinch will do you!). And when a recipe calls for a salad with dressing, stick to the serving size for fats—one tablespoon per person, per salad.

A note on serving sizes: as a rule of thumb, I've designed these portion sizes around guidelines that work for an average-size woman. You may need to adjust the amount of your portions— if you are still hungry, for instance. Again, I don't want you to worry about calories. When you eat in a clean way without extras like sugar or additives to slow down your system, you will naturally arrive at a healthy weight. If you want to lose weight, the most effective way is to follow this eating approach and add more physical activity (you will find more about the benefits of exercise and suggestions for activities in chapter 9).

Serving Sizes

These serving sizes are based on an average-size woman who exercises regularly but not intensely. Depending on your body type, you may need more calories, especially if your frame is bigger and/or you exercise more frequently and for longer durations.

Protein: 3–4 ounces (fish, poultry, pork, bison, lean beef)

Good fats: 1–2 tablespoons (nuts, nut butters, seeds, olive or coconut oil)

Vegetables: 1–2 cups (though you can eat as many vegetables as you wish!)

Grains and legumes: ½ cup (grains, pasta, rice, lentils, beans)

Dairy: ½ cup (milk, yogurt, hard cheese)

Eggs: 1

Tofu: ½ cup

WEEK ONE

Day 1

Breakfast: egg or egg white scramble with sautéed vegetables

Lunch: tomato bisque, cut raw vegetables, and ¼ cup hummus for dipping

Dinner: oven-roasted *Miso-Glazed Salmon; baked sweet potato and side of steamed spinach

Day 2

Breakfast: **organic chicken breakfast sausage

Lunch: grilled or sautéed chicken over broccoli rabe and garlic sautéed in olive oil

Dinner: *Vegetarian Chili with Beans

Day 3

Breakfast: Greek yogurt, walnuts, and flax or chia seed as topping

Lunch: pescatarian Cobb salad: chopped romaine lettuce, red onions, olives, tuna (fresh or canned), and feta crumbles

Dinner: stir-fried vegetables over wild rice or quinoa with a side of sautéed chicken breast

Day 4

Breakfast: poached organic egg over sautéed vegetables

Lunch: *Butternut Squash Soup

Dinner: sautéed shrimp and greens (kale, collards, spinach) over organic polenta

Day 5

Breakfast: steel-cut organic oats with crushed walnuts and a sprinkle of cinnamon

Lunch: **veggie burger over a bed of salad greens

Dinner: roasted or pan-seared salmon or yellowtail; side of arugula and beet salad; side of *Roasted Cauliflower

Day 6

Breakfast: *Avocado Toast (on organic whole-grain or gluten-free bread)

Lunch: *Black Bean Soup

Dinner: steamed arctic char with sautéed broccoli rabe and side of wild rice

Day 7

Breakfast: almond butter on toast (organic whole-grain or gluten-free)

Lunch: grilled shrimp skewers with a side of chopped tomato, cucumber, and red (or yellow) peppers drizzled with a vinegar of your choice (red wine, rice wine, or white wine vinegar, for example).

Dinner: roasted ¼ chicken, chopped cucumber salad, side of *Caesar Salad

WEEK TWO

Day 1

Breakfast: Greek yogurt with crushed nuts and a sprinkle of cinnamon

Lunch: *Roasted Cauliflower with a side of green salad

Dinner: *Miso-Glazed Salmon

Day 2

Breakfast: egg white scramble with salsa

Lunch: *Avocado Salmon Salad—tossed with herbed vinaigrette

Dinner: slow-cooked lentils over cauliflower rice with sautéed dark greens

Day 3

Breakfast: *Green Smoothie

Lunch: *Avocado Toast; cut raw vegetables

Dinner: *Black Bean Soup; barley plus a side of green or chopped salad

Day 4

Breakfast: steel-cut oats with crushed walnuts and a sprinkle of cinnamon

Lunch: grilled shrimp over salad greens with half a small avocado

Dinner: *Vegetarian Chili with Beans

Day 5

Breakfast: poached egg over *Avocado Toast

Lunch: **veggie burger with melted cheese (optional)

Dinner: roasted ¼ chicken and sautéed vegetables and wild rice

Day 6

Breakfast: egg white scramble with vegetarian "sausage"

Lunch: grilled or roasted chicken over salad greens

Dinner: vegetable stir-fry over wild rice, quinoa, or barley

Day 7

Breakfast: tofu or egg scramble with sautéed vegetables

Lunch: tomato bisque with side of *Avocado Toast

Dinner: *Grilled Filet Steak and Arugula

....
WEEK THREE
....

Day 1

Breakfast: egg scramble with salsa

Lunch: *Greek Salad

Dinner: black bean and tempeh tacos with organic corn tortillas and salsa

Day 2

Breakfast: poached egg over black beans

Lunch: chicken soup with wild rice or barley

Dinner: *Vegetarian Chili with Beans; side of chopped salad

Day 3

Breakfast: Greek yogurt with crushed nuts and a sprinkle of cinnamon

Lunch: leftover *Vegetarian Chili with Beans

Dinner: grilled salmon steaks and green salad

Day 4

Breakfast: *Green Smoothie

Lunch: chopped fish salad on whole-grain toast (use pole-caught tuna or try mackerel, sardines, or herring)

Dinner: *Asian Chicken Lettuce Wraps

Day 5

Breakfast: *Goat Cheese Frittata

Lunch: tomato bisque, with a wedge of good sharp cheese

Dinner: **cauliflower-crust cheese pizza

Day 6

Breakfast: steel-cut oats with crushed nuts and sprinkle of cinnamon

Lunch: **veggie burger with a side of green salad or chopped carrots and celery

Dinner: *Farro Risotto with a side of green salad

Day 7

Breakfast: *Avocado Toast

Lunch: turkey or salmon burger over salad greens

Dinner: "breakfast for dinner": *Goat Cheese Frittata

WEEK FOUR

Day 1

Breakfast: *Green Smoothie

Lunch: *Butternut Squash Soup

Dinner: Stir-fried tofu and vegetables over wild rice or quinoa

Day 2

Breakfast: poached egg over whole grain bread/toast

Lunch: chopped vegetable salad with grilled shrimp and avocado

Dinner: *Asian Chicken Lettuce Wraps

Day 3

Breakfast: Greek yogurt with crushed nuts and a sprinkle of cinnamon

Lunch: leftover *Asian Chicken Lettuce Wraps

Dinner: oven-roasted *Miso-Glazed Salmon; baked sweet potato and green salad

Day 4

Breakfast: **chicken breakfast sausage

Lunch: *Greek Salad

Dinner: sautéed shrimp and dark greens with polenta

Day 5

Breakfast: tofu scramble with sautéed greens
Lunch: *Black Bean Soup
Dinner: *Farro Risotto

Day 6

Breakfast: *Green Smoothie
Lunch: *Butternut Squash Soup
Dinner: roasted ¼ chicken or pork loin with wild rice and salad

Day 7

Breakfast: egg white scramble with salsa, side of half an avocado
Lunch: grilled chicken or pork over salad greens sprinkled with almonds or chickpeas
Dinner: roasted or pan-seared tempeh with black beans and wild rice

9

Just a Little Exercise
to Keep You Lively

You may remember the particular joy of running and playing as a child. Racing, leaping, rolling around a backyard, careening through gym class or around the playground, chasing friends around and around a city block, then falling into bed at the end of the day exhausted—but also elated and deeply satisfied. Those feelings aren't limited to childhood. They're also accessible through the power of exercise.

Being physically active does remarkable things for the human body and mind. Exercise prevents disease, transforms mood, boosts sleep, and slows aging. Physical activity keeps hormones in balance and slows their rate of decline with age. Routine exercise is as powerful as medications in treating chronic diseases such as heart disease and diabetes; it lacks medication's side effects and brings many additional benefits. A sedentary lifestyle, on the other hand, accelerates aging and heightens risk for illness and disease, hastening their onset. An absence of physical activity also exacerbates depression and anxiety, undermines sleep, and diminishes energy and vitality. Without regular exercise, it's difficult for many people to maintain a healthy weight.

Making exercise a priority is your responsibility, part of a commitment to caring for yourself and protecting your health and longevity. It is also your right. Time for exercise often gets delayed, curtailed, or altogether lost by busy schedules and other people's needs. Habits of inactivity become entrenched. When you don't have a regular exercise routine, it's easy to forget that exercise feels good and that it's pleasurable to work up a sweat, to feel your body developing strength and endurance. It's also easy to forget that exercise boosts your mood, energy, and cognitive functioning—these are very real, scientifically supported benefits that you don't want to miss out on! Obviously, women who exercise also feel and look more youthful and have more supple skin, a bright complexion, a strong and confident posture, toned muscles, and trim curves.

I am sure you have heard of these many benefits to staying active. I am also sure you don't like to be told what to do. My suggestions for exercise are premised on your discovering or knowing what you enjoy doing. Do you like to walk with friends or your pooch? Do you enjoy dancing to music in a Zumba class, perhaps? Do you prefer solitary workouts at a gym or at home, where you ride a stationary bicycle or follow a yoga routine on a DVD or streamed app on your phone? Are you motivated best when you've signed up for a spin, yoga, Pilates, or ballet barre class and paid for it?

You know what you like. You know what makes you bored. You know what to do. In this chapter, I am offering you some more information to motivate you to incorporate physical activity into your daily life. That's right: it's best for you to move a little every single day. You'll also find some suggestions for types of exercises that you may enjoy, as well as some information to motivate you—the science of exercise is fascinating! If you are already active regularly—wonderful! If you do not have a regular exercise routine or you're feeling a bit rusty, you will find some tips on how to get started incorporating physical activity into your daily life. And keep in mind that you want to incorporate both cardio (to get your heart pumping!) and weight-bearing exercises that strengthen your muscles and skeleton.

Exercise and Your Hormonal Health

Estrogen and exercise influence and reinforce one another. Keeping estrogen levels healthy protects and enhances a woman's ability to be physically active. Estrogen

- Guards against bone loss
- Protects and enhances muscle strength
- Keeps inflammation in check, helping avoid stiffness and pain
- Protects the immune system and promotes tissue healing and postexercise recovery
- Invigorates energy levels

Estrogen is far from the only hormone that enhances your ability to exercise. Overall hormone balance is important to maintaining physical strength and endurance, to protecting and building bone and muscle, and to facilitating neurogenesis. Beyond estrogen, these hormones are particularly effective at increasing your capacity to exercise:

- Testosterone improves overall athletic ability. It protects against and reverses age-related declines in physical skills, including balance, coordination, strength, and endurance. Testosterone helps build bone and muscle. Healthy levels of testosterone—and its enhancements to physical ability and strength—help reduce the frequency and severity of injury.

- Human growth hormone (HGH) enhances your overall ability to exercise and have stamina and helps you maintain your fitness level as you age. *HGH should not be used for excess muscle development beyond your individual natural physiology.*

- DHEA enhances cardiovascular performance. DHEA is critical to acclimation for aerobic exercise at high altitudes. It also increases bone strength and promotes greater muscle mass and muscle strength.

- Regular exercise keeps cortisol levels in check and works like a miracle stress reducer. It also ups endorphins that further help undermine the negative effects of stress.

Exercise and your hormones work together. Your hormone levels, especially estrogen, enable and enhance exercise; in turn, exercise helps keep you in hormonal balance. Indeed, regular exercise slows the decline of estrogen and will help keep you feeling agile and alive.

How Exercise Boosts Your Capacity for Wellness

Science has established a great deal of information about the powerful benefits of exercise to mind and body health—and we continue to learn more about just how profoundly important and health promoting physical exercise is to human life.

Many of the benefits you'll read about below may be familiar to you; some may be new. Until everyone is getting sufficient exercise to help them avoid illness and disease, regulate mood, and slow aging; until we no longer struggle as a society with obesity and metabolic disorders; until we've been untethered from our collective reliance on medications to treat diseases that can be prevented and alleviated by physical activity, the fundamental benefits of exercise warrant being regularly and pointedly repeated.

Pumps Your Heart. Physical activity confers deep benefits to cardiovascular health. Exercise—both cardio and strength training (aerobic and anaerobic exercise)—protects against and reduces arterial sclerosis. Regular exercise lowers blood pressure and helps the heart work more efficiently and effectively to move blood throughout the body. Exercise also reduces risk for stroke.

Deters Cancer. Exercise guards against the development of breast cancer and other cancers, lowering cancer risk for women of all ages. The more you exercise, the lower your risk for dying from cancer, including breast cancer. Vigorous exercise reduces breast cancer risk in healthy-weight women by 30 percent. Exercise decreases the rate of growth and spread of benign breast disease that can precede the development of breast cancer. Breast cancer risk is inversely associated with moderate and vigorous physical activity. For women under the age of fifty, moderate exercise was the factor most strongly linked to reduced breast cancer risk. For women over age fifty, vigorous exercise had the most robust connection to lowering breast cancer risk. For women already diagnosed with breast cancer, maintaining an exercise routine leads to higher survival rates.

Boosts Your Immunity. Moderate exercise provides a boost to the immune system, helping the body ward off illness. Exercise also reduces and limits the rise of stress hormones that interfere with healthy immune function. Physical activity promotes detoxifying processes in the body and increases antioxidant function. Exercise that is too frequent or strenuous can backfire on the immune system, however. Exercising too hard can weaken and undermine immune function.

Fights Inflammation. Moderate exercise can help the body reduce inflammation. Both cardiovascular exercise and strength training at moderate levels contribute to lowering inflammation. While physical exertion typically promotes a temporary increase in the body's inflammatory response, systemic and chronic inflammation decreases with regular moderate exercise. Overtraining and exercising too strenuously, on the other hand, can trigger chronic, unhealthful inflammation.

Supports Your Weight and Metabolism. Exercise in all forms and at all levels of intensity burns calories and can help women maintain a healthy weight or lose weight. Exercise also promotes deep, important changes to metabolic function, helping improve glucose regulation and increase insulin sensitivity, promoting hormone changes that guard against obesity, metabolic disorders, and diabetes. Sedentary women who are postmenopausal who begin to engage in moderate to vigorous exercise show significant changes to their insulin, leptin, and adiponectin levels—all signs of improved metabolic health.

Improves Your Mood. Exercise provides a powerful lift to mood, releasing endorphins that promote feelings of well-being, satisfaction, and confidence. Physical activity boosts production and release of serotonin and of BDNF (brain-derived neurotrophic factor). Exercise can help alleviate depression as effectively or more effectively than antidepressant medications. Exercise helps limit and reduce stress and lowers anxiety. Vigorous exercise is also effective at diminishing panic disorders. The benefits of exercise to mood can be experienced swiftly, often within minutes. There are long-term benefits of regular exercise for mood regulation and for protection against mood disorders.

Helps You Sleep. Being physically active promotes healthy sleep. Exercise improves both sleep quality and duration and promotes additional time in deep or slow-wave sleep, which is the most restorative and rejuvenating phase of sleep for the body. Exercising too close to bedtime can interfere with sleep, so it's best to schedule exercise no closer than three hours before lights-out.

Fortifies Cognition. Exercise improves cognitive performance, including memory and learning, and protects against declines in cognitive function with age. A study of menopausal women ages fifty-nine to sixty-eight showed they increased their cognitive function after three months of regular exercise. Both cardiovascular exercise and strength training enhance memory. Research shows running on a treadmill increases the rate at which the hippocampus creates new brain cells.

The Anti-aging Powers of Exercise

One of the most potent—and alluring—benefits of exercise is its ability to slow the aging process. This anti-aging capacity of exercise not only defers and prevents the development of chronic diseases, from obesity and diabetes to cancer and cardiovascular conditions, it also allows you to age well, to grow older with mental and physical prowess, dexterity, flexibility, and endurance. Exercise—even moderate levels and small amounts of physical activity—extends life span. Specifically, physical exercise improves cellular functioning:

- Exercise stimulates AMPK, an enzyme that regulates cellular metabolism, guarding against diabetes, obesity, weight gain, and physiological degeneration.
- Regular exercise is associated with longer telomeres, the cap-like structures located at the ends of DNA strands that protect DNA from damage. Longer telomeres correspond to increased longevity and lower risk for cancer and other diseases. A recent study shows that athletes have longer telomeres than nonathletes.
- Exercise increases mitochondria in cells; mitochondria are the "energy cells" of our body. Mitochondria also stimulate apoptosis, the programmed death of cells that is one mechanism by which the body avoids the development of cancer.

Think About Exercise in a New Way

Many women dread exercise, especially if they are not accustomed to it. So I ask my patients to think about exercise as a little bit of movement each day. Don't go from zero to sixty. Read through some of the activities described below—you might find one or two that you already enjoy or that spark some interest or curiosity. Give yourself just one simple goal: to come away with a few exercises that you know you can fit into a week.

The timing of exercise and the kind of exercise you do will vary according to your individual preferences, fitness level, and access to a gym or equipment. One woman may love a morning spin class, another a Pilates mat class three times a week. One woman may love the gym, while another feels a strong pull to exercise outdoors. Some women may relish working out with friends or in groups, taking pleasure in the social aspect of exercise, while others may find deep contentment in a solitary run or hike through the woods. I'm less interested in the particular exercise you choose than in making sure that your thinking about exercise becomes more positive.

Here are a few fundamental attitude shifts that I'd like you to consider:

Try to be physically active every day. I recommend trying to do something each day, but not in excess. The most efficient and effective exercise is thirty minutes three times a week. Specifically, it has been shown that thirty minutes of intense interval training three times per week has the most positive effect on health, weight loss, and overall well-being. So take a moment and ask yourself if you can devote a half hour to the broad and lasting benefits of exercise to your health and wellness. That investment of a half hour three days a week suddenly looks like the deal of the century, a fantastically worthwhile use of your time. Exercise can reduce or eliminate reliance on pharmaceutical medications, having been shown as effective (or more so) in treating and lowering mortality for several common chronic diseases, including cardiovascular disease, diabetes, and depression. Think of a daily dose of exercise as your most potent, life-promoting medicine.

Include both cardiovascular and strength activities. A combination of aerobic exercise and anaerobic exercise delivers a full, rounded roster of benefits and protections to a woman's health while also encouraging variety. Particularly for women, who are at significantly greater risk for osteoporosis as they age than men, regular strength-building exercise can help provide protection to bone health and guard against injury and falls. The combination of cardio and strength activities also boosts metabolism and promotes more effective weight loss.

Incorporate variety. Varying forms of exercise and physical activity confers several benefits to a woman's mind and body health and to her ability to sustain a healthy exercise habit. Switching up exercise types keeps both mind and body challenged, prevents boredom, and generally helps avoid the feeling of being in a rut that can arise when doing the same exercise over and over again. Changing it up and varying the types of exercise helps the body remain continually adaptive to new physical challenges, keeping a broad set of physical skills in play and avoiding the plateaus that can arise with repeated sessions of the same physical activity. Research suggests that adding and maintaining variety to exercise patterns may help boost the longevity-promoting benefits of physical activity.

The Benefits of Strength Training (Anaerobic Exercise)

Boosts metabolism, increases calories burned by the body during exercise and daily activities

Increases lean muscle mass

Prevents bone loss, promotes bone growth (increased bone density), reduces risk for osteoporosis

Improves glucose function and lowers blood sugar levels, reducing risk for diabetes

Enhances mood

Reduces arthritic pain

Decreases risks for injury, both exercise-related and non-exercise-related

Enhances coordination and balance

Benefits of Cardio (Aerobic Exercise)

Increases oxygen levels in the blood

Strengthens heart, increases blood flow throughout the body

Lowers blood pressure

Elevates HDL ("good" cholesterol), lowers LDL ("bad" cholesterol)

Reduces risks for diabetes, cardiovascular disease, stroke, cancer

Lowers blood sugar and improves insulin sensitivity

Moves unwanted substances out of tissues, aids in detoxification

Enhances immune system function

Triggers endorphins, which elevate mood, enhance feelings of well-being, alleviate pain, and diminish stress

Helps maintain and increase physical mobility and flexibility

Burns fat and increases lean muscle

A Targeted Workout

A balanced exercise program contains both aerobic exercise (cardio) and anaerobic exercise (strength training), while also addressing the mind-body connection. Aerobic exercise provides conditioning for the cardiovascular and respiratory systems, while anaerobic exercise targets muscle fitness. Both also contribute to bone strength. Together, regular cardio and strength training will improve the body's overall fitness levels, help keep you at a healthy weight, and lower your risk for illness and disease. Many of the workouts I discuss below combine cardio and strength training in a single session.

The mind-body component of exercise is an important element not to be overlooked. Mind-body exercise uses several practices—guided imagery, breathing exercises, mindfulness—to deepen awareness of the body, reduce mental and physical stress and tension, and deepen and enhance breathing.

Again, as you work toward a goal of exercising four to five days a week, start slowly. Perhaps your workout is 15–20 minutes. That's fine. As you become more comfortable (and more fit!), you will more than likely want to sustain your workout longer, gradually reaching 30 or 45 minutes of activity. Ideally, a comprehensive workout will be 45–60 minutes.

If you've not been active recently, you may need to start with less frequent or shorter workouts and build up to this goal. Before you begin, consult with your physician about your health and fitness for exercise, and together decide on an approach that suits your individual needs and challenges.

What Is HIIT?

Now, for a total mind-body challenge that can improve your fitness, accelerate weight loss (if that's your desire), and reset your metabolism, try HIIT, or high-intensity interval training. This approach combines cardio and strength training while varying the intensity of exertion levels. HIIT workouts alternate short periods of vigorous exertion with periods of low to moderate exertion, or active recovery. The bursts of high-intensity effort interspersed with recovery periods provide a highly effective and efficient workout, one that conditions the heart, builds endurance, and strengthens muscles and bones. HIIT workouts are not meant to be long. Rather, they make the most of shorter sessions. Though HIIT workouts are often shorter than traditional workouts, they tend to burn more calories, thanks to the periods of high-intensity exertion. HIIT sessions also prime the body for more postexercise calorie burn than traditional workouts do. HIIT workouts can be tailored to all fitness levels and ages. Each individual works to his or her own level of vigorous exertion and recovery pace of low to moderate exertion. (The American College of Sports Medicine recommends that high-intensity intervals reach 80 percent of an individual's maximum heart rate and that recovery intervals fall within 40–50 percent of maximum heart rate.)

Performed regularly, HIIT delivers excellent conditioning for both the cardiovascular and respiratory systems. The endurance building of HIIT will increase your capacity for exercise and physical activity and also provide you with more energy and stamina throughout the day. The brief periods of intense exercise coax your body into its anaerobic training zone, which powers up the body's metabolism and its ability to burn calories through fat, not muscle. HIIT also stimulates production of the body's own HGH. Here are some ways to get some HIIT!

Take HIIT classes. HIIT classes have become tremendously popular at gyms and fitness centers. Classes such as spinning and Tabata (a form of HIIT circuit training) employ high-intensity interval training to deliver major workout benefits within short sessions. Many HIIT classes will accommodate a wide range of fitness levels. There are also video and streaming HIIT workouts available. Follow these basic guidelines below to create a custom HIIT routine. Check out Dr. Mark J. Smith's method for HIIT! (See docsmith.org.)

Designate 1 minute for each exercise move. For 40 seconds, do as many repetitions of the movement as you can. For the remaining 20 seconds, rest or continue to exercise lightly, such as walking in place.

Put a sequence together. After you've finished the first exercise and rest interval, move on to the next. Create a string of 1-minute moves (40 seconds on, 20 seconds to rest). Ten individual exercises in sequence, repeated 3 times, will provide you with a robust, balanced half-hour HIIT workout. If 30 minutes is too much at first, start with a shorter duration and work toward 15, 20, and eventually 30 minutes as a goal. The same goes for the timing of intervals. If 40 seconds of vigorous movement is overwhelming, scale it back to 30, with 30 seconds of rest.

Target your upper and lower body. If you're putting together your own routine, be sure to include moves that target different parts of the body, including arms and shoulders, thighs, buttocks, and calves. Always engage your core muscles for support and stability and to build core strength.

Turn a regular workout into a HIIT workout. One of the great advantages of HIIT is its adaptability. Almost any workout can be converted into a HIIT workout by including periodic intervals of vigorous exertion, such as sprinting, into an otherwise moderate workout. Creating HIIT workouts from forms of exercise you're already doing is a great way to begin to incorporate HIIT into your exercise routine. Some of the most common workouts that can become HIIT sessions are:

Walking
Jogging
Swimming
Cycling
Hiking
Rowing
Stair stepping/elliptical training

To convert these popular workouts to HIIT sessions, simply add periodic bursts of vigorous exertion. If you're running, sprint for 30 seconds and run in recovery mode for 4–5 minutes before sprinting again. A swim or a cycle can become a HIIT workout using the same basic formula: 30 seconds of moving as vigorously as you can through the exercise, alternating with 4–5 minutes of low to moderate effort.

Another advantage of HIIT? It's highly portable. You don't need lots of equipment—you can use your body's own weight to build strength and raise your heart rate. Adding some simple equipment, such as hand weights and a jump rope, can expand your HIIT options. It's also not necessary to engage in complicated routines. Simple moves that are already familiar to many active women can be combined into a HIIT workout you can do anywhere—your living room, a hotel room, your vacation cabin.

If you're already working out and familiar with common exercise moves, you may feel ready to jump right in and create your own HIIT workout. If you're not familiar with these exercises, I recommend scheduling a few sessions with a trainer, who can help you learn the proper methods and form for these or other moves.

A few words of caution: some classes and other HIIT-influenced workouts take the valuable, effective exercise strategy of HIIT to an unhealthful extreme. An hour of nonstop, frantic cycling is not a HIIT workout—it's sixty minutes of overexertion that can damage your body and undermine your health. Make sure you're working out for thirty minutes, no more—even if that means leaving class early. (Better yet, find a HIIT class that doesn't exceed thirty minutes.)

As always, listen to your body and don't push yourself to overdo the vigorous intervals of HIIT or to skimp on the rest intervals. Keep in mind what vigorous exertion feels like and also what moderate and low exertion feel like. Remember, your exercise should leave you feeling energized, not exhausted and depleted.

Common Exercises For HIIT

Lunges: front, side, and back

Squats

Push-ups, traditional and modified

High knee steps

Butt kicks

Jumping jacks

Mountain climbers

Planks

Bicycle crunches

Biceps curls

Triceps dips

Shadowboxing

Jumping rope

Tone and Strengthen

These workouts also often combine cardio and strength training, but without the bursts of vigorous exercise of HIIT. These exercises can engage you at low to moderate or even vigorous exertion, raising your heart rate and providing conditioning for your cardiovascular system. They also will work both large and small muscle groups, helping create muscle that is long, lean, and toned while also building bone strength and promoting flexibility.

Some forms of exercise, such as yoga, place particular attention on the mind-body connection. Bear in mind that any exercise can be a mind-body exercise when you incorporate attention to breathing, awareness of the body, and a gentle, mindful focus on your thoughts, feelings, and sensations in the present moment.

Yoga. With its emphasis on building total-body strength and enhancing flexibility, yoga is an excellent regular component of a woman's exercise routine at any age. Yoga promotes mindfulness, helps flush the body of toxins, improves breathing, and promotes stress reduction. There are many varieties of yoga out there, some more physically rigorous than others. A good instructor can help you develop a practice suited to your individual fitness needs and goals.

Pilates. Pilates is a guided routine of exercises that develop the body's core strength, as well as muscles in the upper and lower body. Like yoga, Pilates can improve flexibility, as well as overall muscle tone and development. Pilates emphasizes breathing, mindfulness, and a deepening awareness of the body.

Tai chi. An ancient form of Chinese martial art, tai chi is a powerful mind-body practice that combines slow, deliberate physical movement with deep breathing and mindfulness. Tai chi helps build muscle strength and flexibility, improves balance, and can provide some aerobic benefit as well.

Walking or jogging. A brisk walk or a light jog elevates the heart rate and tones muscles, especially in the lower body. These workouts also contribute to muscle joint flexibility. Women who enjoy running should absolutely do so. Be aware, however, that running is hard on your joints, especially the lower back and knees, and can lead to overexertion and overtraining. It's wonderful to challenge your body and mind through fitness training, but only to a point. Light to moderate running delivers greater health benefits and less risk of injury and the negative effects of overexertion than extremely fast-paced or very long runs. Walking confers nearly all the benefits of running without exposing the body to the risks of injury and overtraining. If you run, do so outdoors or on a treadmill. You can turn a walk or a run into a hike by climbing a hill outdoors, by raising the incline on the treadmill, or by using the elliptical or stair-stepper training machines.

Dance. These exhilarating workouts provide total body benefits. They improve coordination, balance, and flexibility. Dancing engages several muscle groups at once and builds overall fitness levels, toning and strengthening muscles and elevating heart rate. The combination of movement and music can be mentally and emotionally uplifting, delivering powerful sensations of freedom and release. There are so many options available if you want to incorporate dance into your exercise routine. Afro-Caribbean, Latin, hip-hop cardio, and ballet barre are among the many types enjoyed by the women I see in my practice.

Swimming. Swimming is a terrific total-body conditioning and strengthening workout for women of all ages and fitness levels. Swimming builds and tones muscles in the upper and lower body and delivers a strong cardiovascular workout—all at very low impact to the body. It can be especially useful for women with back and knee issues or women with muscle and joint pain and stiffness, including women with arthritis and fibromyalgia.

Take Time to Recover

Recovery and rest are essential to a balanced exercise regimen and to protecting health and preventing injury. I understand the temptation to push harder and the desire to progress quickly toward fitness goals. Yet many of my patients report having their best workouts after their rest day. This comes as no surprise to me. Rest days don't get in the way of progress; rather, they fuel it.

Commit to your rest days and to finding some time every day to relax and recharge.

Longer and faster exercise isn't always better. Overtraining, whether exercising too often or pushing oneself too hard, can cause stress and damage to the body. Extreme exertion breaks down the body's ability to repair itself and can even damage DNA. Also, the older we get, the more vulnerable we are to the damaging effects of very vigorous exercise. This doesn't mean that you should avoid breaking a sweat, but do pay attention to your body's signals about the impact exercise is having on your body and mind. Avoiding too-vigorous exercise and overtraining helps avert injury, and you heal faster from injuries if you exercise moderately. Maintaining moderation and balance in your exercise enables you to sustain a regular routine—week in, week out and over the course of a life span. Keeping up with consistent exercise as you age slows the aging process and protects against disease.

The signs of overtraining:

- Muscle pain and stiffness that lasts for hours or days after a workout, and may be intense
- Fatigue after a workout that persists throughout the day and perhaps into the next
- Feeling as though you need a nap after an exercise session
- Coming down more frequently with colds and flu and taking longer to recover
- Difficulty and diminished ability performing daily tasks

How Strenuous Is Too Strenuous?

When figuring out what you enjoy doing for physical exercise, you'll likely hear physicians or fitness experts talk about different levels of exercise intensity—moderate exercise, vigorous exercise, light exercise. Do you know how to gauge physical exertion?

Light exercise: Exercising lightly is considered exertion slightly beyond a normal resting state. Examples of light physical activity for most people include slow or leisurely walking, light cleaning, gardening, and any other activities that require standing and some movement for fifteen to twenty minutes—even a little bit of movement counts!

Moderate exercise: Moderate physical exertion involves more pronounced changes to the body. When you exercise moderately, the heart rate is elevated and a person may sweat lightly. Breathing becomes more rapid and pronounced, but it's still possible for most people to hold a conversation. Brisk walking, cycling at a light or slow pace, swimming leisurely, yoga, Pilates, light circuit training, and strength training are examples of moderate exercise.

Vigorous exercise: Exercise at a vigorous level of intensity elevates the heart rate significantly. Sweating is steady and can be profuse. Breathing is rapid and heavy—during vigorous exercise, it can be difficult to have a conversation or speak more than a few words at a time. Running, hiking at a fast pace or up a steep hill, swimming, high-intensity circuit or interval workouts that combine cardio and strength training, and spinning are all forms of vigorous exercise that will get your heart pumping and your fat burning.

Keep in mind that any and all levels of exercise are valuable and contribute to your health and well-being. For people who are moving into a new exercise routine after being sedentary, you might want to take things slowly—starting with a low or moderate level of exertion. Whatever your level of fitness, it's important to balance challenging yourself with listening to your body and paying attention to the signs it is sending you about your exertion levels. Exercise at the right level of intensity should make you feel invigorated, not drained.

Metabolic energy equivalent, or MET, is a method used by scientists and fitness experts to measure physical exertion. One MET is the amount of energy a person requires just to be awake and alert, resting quietly. Exercise intensity with MET is measured by how much more energy the activity requires than this resting baseline.

Light exercise: 1–3 MET
Moderate exercise: 3–6 MET
Vigorous exercise: more than 6 MET

MET can be a useful tool in assessing exertion, but it's neither comprehensive nor perfect. MET levels do not take into account age, fitness level, or other individual factors that make significant contributions to exercise's impact and difficulty. A moderate workout in MET terms for one individual may be a vigorous workout for another. MET can be a useful guideline in many cases, such as when attempting to distinguish between a moderate workout and a vigorous one. But the most important gauge is the body's own response to physical exertion.

Eating and Snacking When You're Active

It's natural to experience an increase in your appetite when you begin to exercise regularly or when you increase the amount and frequency of exercise in your routine. The trick is not to let your hunger undermine the good that exercise can do in helping manage weight. I've seen many of my patients enthusiastically dive in to a new exercise regimen, eagerly anticipating both the health benefits and the weight loss they expect to receive—only to feel deeply discouraged a few months later when they've put on weight, not lost it. There are ways to handle the hunger that may arise when you boost your exercise levels so you can derive the deepest, fullest benefits from your hard work.

Don't reward yourself with food. It can be tempting to give yourself some leeway to indulge in "treat" foods as a reward for working out. But this habit detracts from the rewards that exercise itself offers to your health and weight. Using food as a reward, even for exercise, isn't a good idea. Find other ways to treat yourself for making the effort to exercise. Think about what relaxes you—a long hot soak in the tub? An hour with a cup of tea and a good book?—and reward yourself accordingly. Even better, take exercise, and the time you spend being physically active, as its own reward, and pay attention to your body getting stronger, more fit, and more limber.

Snack smart. Planning for your hunger before it strikes will help you avoid making unhealthful choices. The right preworkout snack will fuel your activity, not slow you down. Eating after you've exercised can help you avoid the deep hunger that often sends us in search of all the "wrong" sorts of foods—sugary treats, salty and starchy snacks. The right combination of lean protein, high-nutrient carbohydrates, and healthy fats consumed in snacks between meals will help keep your blood sugar even and stimulate hormones (ghrelin) that induce feelings of fullness.

Supplements to Maximize Your Exercise Results

A diet of healthful, unprocessed whole foods in moderation helps prepare the body to be physically active. High-quality nutritional supplements can further support a woman's ability to exercise regularly, increasing her capacity for physical exertion and promoting swift and full recovery from both injury and exercise's regular wear and tear on the body. By taking the recommended amounts of these supplements, you can enhance the results of your regular exercise routine:

Vitamin D

D-ribose

Quercetin

L-carnitine

Theanine

L-glutamine

Rhodalia—herb

Planning Your Week of Exercise

How you set up your weekly workout routine will depend on your particular schedule and obligations. I encourage my patients to make time in their schedule to exercise in the morning. Morning exercise provides a potent energy boost and fires up the body's metabolism. It also gets the day's exercise on the books before the rest of life gets in the way. Job and family responsibilities may make regular morning workouts unrealistic. If you can schedule one or two a week, great. If all your workouts need to happen at lunch or in the evening, that's perfectly okay. One of the keys to sticking with an exercise regimen is to schedule your workout sessions with a realistic eye for how your daily life unfolds.

A similar principle holds for the days of the week you work out. Ideally, you'd work out two to three days in a row, take a rest day, and resume for another couple days of more intense physical activity. If your commitments to work and family make this schedule difficult, opt for a schedule of five days on, two days off—or whatever weekly routine or rhythm suits you. Some people find it's helpful to align their five days of exercise with the Monday–Friday workweek.

If you haven't exercised in a while, it's best for you to start slowly. You may also want to check with your physician or health care provider so that you choose a routine that is both realistic and safe. It's easy to injure yourself if you suddenly go from zero or sixty. If this is the case, I have noted adjustments you can make so that you can introduce exercise and gradually build up your level of intensity. For instance, if you have not been exercising and feel a bit out of shape, don't jump right into a HIIT routine. Instead, begin with walking regularly for twenty to thirty minutes four or five times a week. Your body will adjust in one or two weeks, and then you may feel ready to try a more intense form of cardio . . . or not. Regardless of your starting point, you can always benefit from doing some strengthening with light weights, as well as including gentle stretches and ten to fifteen minutes of mindfulness as a way to rest and restore.

Take a look at the weeklong plan below and read through the suggestions to see what activities appeal to you and what schedule is realistic for you, and then carve out time to make it happen!

A WEEK AT A GLANCE

	Sunday	Monday	Tuesday	Wednesday	Thursday	Friday	Saturday
Exercise Type	Rest & Restore: meditation, walking meditation	30-minute walk; jog; spin; swim; Tabata; or other HIIT class	Strengthen & Stretch: yoga, Pilates, barre, tai chi, or at-home stretches with light weights	30-minute walk; jog; spin; swim; Tabata; or other HIIT class	Strengthen & Stretch: yoga, Pilates, barre, tai chi, or at-home stretches with light weights	30-minute walk; jog; spin; swim; Tabata; or other HIIT class	Do something different: hike, bike ride; dance, or other leisure activity

YOUR HEALTH JOURNAL: TRACK YOUR ACTIVITY

Use your journal to record your exercise. Write down the time and day and the type of exercise. You might even want to jot down what you liked and what you'd prefer to skip. These notes will help you stay motivated and in tune with yourself and keep your exercise routine in the forefront of your mind and your priorities. As you plan your exercise for the week, make sure you write down specific days when you rest and restore your body. For example, if you've had a day of an intense HIIT workout, then follow it with a day of no workout. If, however, you walked and did yoga one day, followed with another day of light exercise (a bike ride or some gardening), then you might not need a full rest day. Listen to what your body is telling you and trust it.

- 3 out of 4 women who wore bras 24 hours a day
- 1 out of 7 women who wore bras more than 12 hours, but not to bed
- 1 out of 168 women who rarely or never wore bras

So am I telling you to burn your bra? Not really. But you can choose to be more aware and perhaps curtail wearing one for more than eight to ten hours a day. Of course, bra use is personal. As with all my patients, my goal is to provide you with the scientific facts about the risks of bra wearing so that you can make informed choices about whether and how often to use them.

If you're like my patients, you're likely concerned about two effects of aging—sagging breasts and pain or discomfort in the breasts. Many women, especially women with large breasts, worry about sagging as a consequence of leaving their bras behind. In fact, the opposite appears to be true. Research demonstrates that bras themselves contribute to increased breast sagging. From what I observe in my patients, bras—especially bras with underwire and other constricting features—may keep the muscles that support the breast from working optimally. I also observe in my patients posture changes that occur when they stop wearing bras—less slouching, more standing up straight, which aids in avoiding sagging and the appearance of sagging.

Before giving up or limiting bra use, many women wonder about pain or discomfort to breasts themselves or to other areas of the body. It's been my observation that women adapt quickly, easily, and without pain or discomfort when they wear bras less frequently. In fact, bra wearing is responsible for aches and pains in the shoulders and back that are resolved when women stop wearing bras. Research shows that shoulder pain also decreases in women as their bra use diminishes.

So what should you wear instead?

Nothing, if that's comfortable. However, there are garments that are safe alternatives to constricting bras. Strapless bandeau tops are a healthy alternative to bras, and they are comfortable for many women. The right garment is one that doesn't exert pressure on the chest wall the way a traditional bra's straps, clasps, and underwire do.

A Breast Massage

A breast massage is a simple and yet incredibly effective way to maintain the elasticity and health of breast tissue. By doing ten to twenty small clockwise and counterclockwise circles while also stimulating your nipples once a day, you greatly enhance the tissue of the breast.

Reducing Chemicals and Toxins in Food

Eating, cooking, purchasing, and storing food are rife with opportunities for unhealthful exposure to chemicals. But you can reduce that exposure with some basic knowledge and commitment to eating well and sourcing healthful foods.

- My first, basic suggestion: buy organic. Investment in your personal food supply is one of the best ways you can decrease your exposure to pesticides, herbicides, and other chemicals. You should also limit dairy and meat, especially red meat and processed meat.
- Try to avoid canned foods and swap out plastic for glass or stainless steel containers for storage.
- Switch from nonstick cooking pans to stainless steel, iron, ceramic, or glass.

- Do not use plastic wrap or aluminum foil.
- Avoid the use of plastic cups, dishes, or flatware.
- Make sure that your drinking water is filtered or purified.

Reducing Exposure in Household Products and Personal Care Products

Our bodies are constantly exposed to chemicals through the environment. Toxins and pollutants are in food, in water, and in the products we come into contact with at work. Products women use every day to clean and care for their bodies are an often overlooked source of chemical exposure. These sources in everyday life contribute to a heavy toxic load and to constant interference with natural estrogen levels and overall hormone function and balance. This everyday exposure triggers physiological dysfunction throughout the body and is a catalyst for disease. Unfortunately, the pervasive presence of xenoestrogens, persistent organic pollutants, and other toxic substances in our environment and in our food and drinking supply mean that none of us can avoid toxic exposure altogether. Nonetheless, you have a number of ways to meaningfully reduce the degree of chemical exposure in your daily life and to reduce the burden of toxins on the body and its delicate, complex endocrine system.

Antiperspirants and Deodorants

Sweat is natural and necessary, a critical physiological function. Sweating flushes the body of toxins. It helps regulate body temperature and promotes circulation. Sweating cleans and purifies skin, clearing dirt, bacteria, and other substances from pores. Sweating that occurs at the underarms helps rid tissues of the breast and surrounding areas of unhealthful, unwanted substances, including toxins. The practice of routinely trying to inhibit sweating and stop the odor associated with underarm sweating is danger-ous to breast health and to health in general. By using deodorants and antiperspirants, we are not only stopping a natural process that's essential to ridding the body of waste and toxins but also introducing chemicals that are actively harmful to the body, espe-cially when applied to the sensitive areas under the arm and on and around the breast.

The chemical additives in antiperspirants and deodorants are absorbed by the skin. Once inside the tissues of the body, many behave like estrogens. Applying chemicals to the skin areas around the breast has a significant estrogenic effect on breast and surround-ing tissues. Breast cancer is more likely to develop in the upper and outer quadrants of the breast, where antiperspirants and deodorants are applied (along with other personal care products such as lotions, creams, cosmetics, and sunscreen).

These products also commonly contain parabens, a form of preservative used widely in deodorants, antiperspirants, lotions, makeup, and sunscreen. Parabens are estrogen-mimicking in the body and have been found in breast cancer tissue.

I recommend against using antiperspirant of any kind. If you are concerned with body odor, use an organic product that does not contain ammonia, phthalates, fragrance, or any other chemical additive. A few good brands include EO, Tom's of Maine, Ursa Major, Schmidt's, and Soapwalla. Many of these products can be found at natural food stores, Whole Foods, or online through Amazon or Thrive Market.

I also urge you not to apply any substance—lotion, gel, perfume, sunscreen, or makeup—to the underarm area or the breast itself. A natural, chemical-free soap and water are fine to use for cleaning these areas. Avoid lathering products—soap, gels, or lotions—that may introduce unwanted chemicals. Pure, minimally processed, and chemical-free soap is safe and the best choice. If you're concerned about odor, apply perfume or scented oils to the underside of the arm along the biceps or to the side of the torso. Just be sure that these products are applied where they do not have direct contact with the underarm or breast areas—this includes the areas of skin above and to the side of the breasts.

Personal Care Products

Chemical toxins and xenoestrogens are in nearly all personal care products that we use daily on our bodies. By avoiding these products, whether by opting to go without or by using safe alternatives, you can avoid the damage and disruption that these chemicals, many of which are xenoestrogens, do to health and hormone balance.

When choosing these products, be sure to select only products with natural ingredients. Avoid products touted as "antibacterial"— they're likely to contain a chemical that mimics and disrupts natural estrogen. Make sure products that contain fragrances are scents derived only from natural sources. A good rule of thumb is this: if you wouldn't eat or cook with an ingredient, you ought not apply it to your body.

This applies to tampons as well. Women and only a few other mammals evolved to have menstrual cycles, and human girls and women are the only species with a fairly substantial flow. So when it comes to tampons, it's crucial that you use organic tampons. Why would you want to insert a chemicalized material into your vagina when you are bleeding? You absorb too many chemicals that could be toxic to your entire body.

Swap out chemical-laden versions of the following products with organic, nontoxic, natural alternatives:

- Shampoo, conditioners
- Cleansing and lathering soaps

- Makeup
- Lotions for shaving, moisturizing
- Sunscreen
- Toothpaste
- Mouthwash and other oral rinses

By swapping out conventional, chemical-laden versions of these common products in favor of natural, nontoxic versions, you reduce your exposure to xenoestrogens and other toxins damaging to the body. Look for products with natural ingredients only, including:

- Household cleaning products
- Dish liquid
- Dishwasher detergent
- Surface cleaners
- Floor and carpet cleaners
- Laundry detergents

The Hazards of Antibacterial Agents

When you see a soap or cleaning product labeled "antibacterial," does it make you reach for that product on the shelf? Does it give you a sense of comfort to think about eradicating unwanted bacteria with a squirt of the bottle or a swipe of a washcloth? These products that promote themselves as antibacterial agents usually contain chemical additives that do far more harm than good. Triclosan and triclocarbon are among the most common chemical disinfectants added to personal care and household products to kill bacteria and fungi. These chemicals are added to soaps, household cleaners, toothpaste and mouthwash, cookware, toys, and even clothing. Triclosan is highly disruptive to endocrine function and hormone balance. It both mimics and disrupts estrogen, and it also disrupts and alters other hormones, including thyroid hormone and testosterone. There is evidence that triclosan and other similar chemicals are disruptive to the immune system. This antibacterial and antifungal chemical agent also aids in the rise of bacteria that are resistant to antibiotics. To avoid this estrogen-mimicking chemical, steer clear of antibacterial soaps and other products for your body and your home. Use simple, natural, nontoxic, minimally processed cleansers to clean your body and your environment.

Keep in Mind the Body's Natural Detox Powers.

The wide proliferation of environmental hazards can feel overwhelming when you're learning about it. It is sobering and frightening to think of all the chemical agents to which we, and our children and grandchildren, are routinely exposed. I ask you not to give in to the temptation to give up. The difficult truth is that none of us can fully protect ourselves from or avoid the toxins that pervade our air, water, and food. But there are many ways you can reduce your exposure to environmental toxins and xenoestrogens, thereby limiting the damage they can do to your health.

Reducing individual exposure to chemical toxins is important to hormonal health and will also reduce your risk of developing other diseases. You can be proactive and support your hormonal health with these strategies:

· **Exercise**: Physical activity boosts the immune system, aids detoxification through sweat, and supports estrogen and hormone balance.

- **Diet**: Avoiding processed foods and limiting meat and dairy products and canned goods reduces direct exposure to toxins. Eat healthfully and maintain a supplement regimen to support immune system function and to bolster the body's ability to guard against disease and respond to environmental toxins and chemical threats.
- **Sleep**: Sleep is a powerful restorer of the body's systems, including the rejuvenation of the immune system.
- **Stress management**: Limiting stress protects the body's ability to ward off disease and foreign agents, including chemical toxins from the environment.

All women are gifted with a bright mind and intelligent body. If you feed your body with simple, organic, nonchemicalized foods and healthful supplements, you will be rewarded with health and vibrancy. Your body will operate more efficiently and for longer without decline. Remember, you have the right to feel good in your body—regardless of your age. And now you have the information to be able to do that!

A Final Note

My dear readers, please know that I think of each and every one of you as a patient. I hope this book has been helpful in opening your eyes and minds to the almost miraculous outcomes so many women have experienced using bioidentical hormone therapy. I wish the same for you. Regardless of your age, background, or hometown, you can with confidence connect with a health care practitioner who will guide you to make the information in this book a part of your life and health.

I also want to reassure you that you can reach out to me directly through my website for any questions you might have.

Resources

BREAKFAST RECIPES

Avocado Toast

This healthy yet deliciously satisfying dish can be enjoyed for breakfast or lunch! If you're looking for a more substantial meal, add a poached egg on top!

Ingredients

½ large avocado or 1 small avocado

½ teaspoon lemon or lime juice

1–2 slices multigrain bread

Coarse sea salt and black pepper to taste or paprika

Directions

1. Peel, pit, and gently mash avocado and squeeze lemon or lime to taste.

2. Meanwhile, toast bread.

3. Spread avocado on toast, sprinkling on salt and pepper or paprika.

Green Smoothie

Ingredients

½ cup fruit of your choice (Research fruits and their sugar content to choose wisely when adding fruit to a smoothie!)

½ cup unsweetened almond or oat milk

¼ cup (or small handful) baby spinach

¼ small avocado

1 tablespoon chia seed (or combination of chia and flaxseed)

Directions

Blend ingredients in a blender for 1–2 minutes.

Goat Cheese Frittata

I love this frittata for breakfast, lunch, or dinner! It's easy to prepare and offers an array of flavors. It also warms up beautifully for leftovers.

Ingredients

2 tablespoons olive oil

3 shallots, diced

8 large eggs (for two or three people)

¾ teaspoon sea salt

¼ teaspoon coarse ground black pepper

1 handful fresh baby spinach

1 cup goat cheese, crumbled or cut into small cubes

Directions

1. Preheat oven to 350°F.
2. In a cast iron or other ovenproof skillet, heat the oil and shallots, cooking until soft and golden.
3. Crack eggs into a bowl and whisk, seasoning with salt and pepper.
4. Pour egg mixture into skillet and stir together with shallots.
5. Gently stir spinach leaves into the egg mixture until wilted.
6. Top the egg mixture with the goat cheese, place in the oven, and bake for 15–20 minutes.

SOUPS AND SIDE RECIPES
· ·

Roasted Butternut Squash Soup

This smooth, rich soup makes for a wonderful fall or winter meal. You can roast the squash the day before you plan to enjoy the soup.

Ingredients

2 tablespoons olive oil

1 cup white or yellow onion, chopped

1 cup celery, chopped

1 cup carrots, chopped

3–4 cups butternut squash (approximately one butternut squash), peeled, quartered, and roasted until soft

Salt and pepper

Cinnamon and/or nutmeg, to taste

1 quart organic vegetable or chicken broth

Directions

1. In a large skillet, heat the oil and then add the onion, celery, and carrots, sautéeing until tender.
2. Add the chunks of butternut squash gradually until all is melded together. Add in salt and pepper and other spices, to taste.
3. Let simmer for 10–15 minutes, and remove from heat before any squash browns.
4. Let cool for 10 minutes.
5. Scoop two cups of mixture at a time into blender and blend with broth until mixture becomes creamy. Add more broth if necessary.
6. Reheat and serve immediately or let cool and then refrigerate to enjoy later.

Roasted Cauliflower

Ingredients

1 head cauliflower, cut into bite-size florets

2 tablespoons olive oil

Pinch of salt

½ teaspoon fresh garlic, minced (or use powder)

½ teaspoon turmeric

Directions

1. Preheat oven to 425°F.
2. In a bowl, toss the cauliflower with olive oil, salt, garlic, and turmeric until evenly coated.
3. Transfer cauliflower to a baking sheet and roast for 30–35 minutes, or until the cauliflower is tender and slightly browned.

Black Bean Soup

Ingredients

1 medium onion, diced

2 cloves garlic, minced

1 red bell pepper, diced

¼ cup water, plus more if needed

1 teaspoon cumin

½ teaspoon smoked paprika

½ teaspoon salt

4 cups cooked black beans (or about 2.5 non-BPA, cans, rinsed and drained)

14.5 ounces tomato, chopped (boxed, canned or fresh)

3 cups organic vegetable broth, plus another cup if desired

Directions

1. In a soup pot over medium heat, cook the onion, garlic, and bell pepper in oil and ¼ cup water until softened, about 5–6 minutes. Add water as necessary to prevent vegetables from sticking.
2. Add the cumin, paprika, and salt and cook for another minute or two until the spices are fragrant.
3. Add black beans, tomatoes, and 3 cups of vegetable broth and bring to a boil.
4. Reduce heat to medium-low and simmer 15–20 minutes.
5. In a blender, puree 2–3 cups of soup at a time.
6. Reheat before serving.

Optional Garnishes

Diced avocado

Sliced green onion

Crushed organic tortilla chips

Vegan sour cream

SALAD RECIPES

· · · · · · · · · · · · · · · · · · ·

Caesar Salad

A Caesar salad is an easy-to-prepare classic, and the ingredients are simple. The dressing is light and flavorful and does not require any hard-to-find ingredients. You can add a protein topping, such as grilled organic chicken or salmon, if desired.

Ingredients
Salad

2 heads organic romaine lettuce, chopped (enough for 2–4 servings)

Parmesan cheese, shredded or shaved

Salt and pepper, to taste

Dressing

¼ teaspoon garlic, minced

1 teaspoon Dijon mustard

1 teaspoon Worcestershire sauce

½ teaspoon lemon juice

1 tablespoon red wine vinegar

1–2 tablespoons olive oil

Directions

1. Combine dressing ingredients in a small bowl and let stand for 2–3 minutes.
2. Whisk oil into dressing until emulsified.
3. To make the salad, toss the lettuce with the dressing and top with the Parmesan cheese.
4. Season with salt and pepper.

Avocado Salmon Salad

This salad is tasty and filling and can be eaten for lunch or dinner.

Ingredients
Salmon

2–4 salmon fillets, boneless and skinless

1 teaspoon garlic salt

⅛ teaspoon pepper

1 teaspoon cilantro, chopped

½ tablespoon olive oil

1 tablespoon lemon juice (freshly squeezed or from bottle)

Salad

1 medium head romaine lettuce (or 4 cups chopped)

½ cucumber, thinly sliced

½ small red onion (½ cup), thinly sliced

5 radishes, thinly sliced

2 avocados, pitted, peeled, and sliced

Lemon-Dill Dressing

3 tablespoons lemon juice

3 tablespoons olive oil

1 teaspoon pink Himalayan sea salt

2 tablespoons fresh dill, chopped

Directions

1. In a small bowl, whisk together dressing ingredients and set aside.
2. To prepare the salmon, season both sides of each fillet with 1 teaspoon garlic salt and ⅛ teaspoon pepper, cilantro, olive oil, and lemon.
3. Bring olive oil to medium heat in a skillet (2–3 minutes), add salmon, and cook 3–4 minutes on each side, or until cooked through (cooking time will vary depending on thickness of salmon fillet).
4. Transfer salmon to a plate and spoon 1 teaspoon of the dressing over each fillet. Set aside to cool to room temperature.
5. Arrange salad ingredients on top (or to side) of salmon in a bowl, layering lettuce, cucumber, red onion, radishes, and avocados.
6. Top with dressing to taste.

Greek Salad

I love Greek salads because of their mix of salt, tang, and a touch of sweet. This is another salad that can benefit from an added protein of your choice—tuna (to give it a niçoise flavor), chicken (making it a bit more American!), or salmon.

Ingredients

1 cucumber, cut into small chunks or sliced

1 green pepper, cut into small chunks or sliced

1 red bell pepper, cut into small chunks or sliced

1 large ripe tomato, cut into eighths

1 medium red onion, thinly sliced

¼ pound feta cheese (soft or hard), cut into triangles (approximately ⅛-inch thick)

½ cup kalamata olives (with pits!)

Olive oil

Red or white wine vinegar

Salt and pepper, to taste

Directions

Place the salad ingredients in a large bowl and dress with olive oil and red or white wine vinegar; season with salt and pepper.

MAIN DISH RECIPES

Miso-Glazed Salmon

This is a flavorful seafood dish that is packed with nutrients! You can enjoy it hot immediately after preparing it or as cold leftovers the next day. (Adapted from Food Network)

Ingredients

¼ cup white miso

2–3 tablespoons low-sodium soy sauce

2 tablespoons rice vinegar

2 tablespoons green onions, minced

1½ tablespoons fresh ginger, minced

2 teaspoons toasted sesame oil

4 salmon fillets, 8 ounces each

Salt and ground pepper, to taste

Directions

1. Place miso, soy sauce, vinegar, onions, ginger, and sesame oil in a large mixing bowl and whisk together.
2. Place salmon fillets in the bowl and marinate for 20 minutes.

3. Meanwhile, heat grill (to about 400 degrees) or skillet.

4. Cook salmon skin side down for 5–7 minutes per side, or until cooked through.

Vegetarian Chili with Beans

Ingredients

1 tablespoon olive oil

1 cup onion, chopped

¾ cup carrots, chopped

3 cloves garlic, minced

1 cup green bell pepper, chopped

1 cup red bell pepper, chopped

¾ cup celery, chopped

1 tablespoon chili powder

1½ cups mushrooms, chopped

1 (28 ounce) box whole peeled tomatoes with liquid, chopped

1 (19 ounce) box or non-BPA can kidney beans with liquid

1 tablespoon ground cumin

1½ teaspoons cilantro, chopped

Directions

1. Heat oil in a large saucepan over medium heat and sauté onions, carrots, and garlic until tender.

2. Stir in green pepper, red pepper, celery, and chili powder. Cook until vegetables are tender, about 6 minutes.

3. Stir in mushrooms and cook 4 minutes.

4. Stir in tomatoes and beans and season with cumin and cilantro.

5. Bring to a boil and reduce heat to medium. Cover and simmer for 20 minutes, stirring occasionally.

Farro Risotto

Farro is an Italian grain that is gaining popularity for its nutty flavor, high fiber, and delicious nutritiousness—all packed into one grain! In this recipe, I've adapted flavor and steps from a recipe created by Yotam Ottolenghi. You can add avocado and greens as a garnish and make this a salad or roasted cauliflower for a more robust main dish.

Ingredients

4 tablespoons olive oil

1 onion, chopped

3 cloves garlic, chopped

1 cup pearled farro

1 pint crushed tomatoes

3–4 cups water

Pinch of lemon zest

½ teaspoon smoked paprika

½ teaspoon dried thyme

2 cups hard feta, chopped or crumbled

Directions

1. In large pan, heat the oil and sauté the onion and garlic until translucent.
2. Add farro to the pan and coat with the mixture.
3. Over medium heat, add tomatoes and 1 cup of water; stir so mixture begins to thicken.
4. Continue to add a cup of water at a time, stirring occasionally.
5. As water is absorbed and farro softens to a chewy consistency, add lemon zest, paprika, and thyme.
6. Right before serving, gently stir feta into risotto.

Asian Chicken Lettuce Wraps

Ingredients

Chicken

2 cups white chicken, cooked and chopped

1 cup chopped mandarin oranges with no sugar added (optional)

2 stalks celery, diced

½ cup carrots, shredded

1 cup purple cabbage, finely shredded or chopped

2 green onions, thinly sliced

½ teaspoon salt

¼ teaspoon coarse black pepper

¼ cup chopped cilantro

1 large Boston or Bibb lettuce

Sesame Ginger Dressing
⅓ cup rice vinegar
¼ cup soy sauce
3 tablespoons sesame seeds
1 tablespoon brown sugar
2 teaspoons fresh ginger, grated
1 garlic clove, grated
1½ teaspoons sesame oil

Directions
1. Whisk dressing ingredients together in a small bowl and set aside.
2. In a large bowl, combine chicken, mandarin oranges (if using), celery, carrots, cabbage, green onions, salt, and pepper. Add ½ cup of dressing and toss to combine.
3. To serve, place a half to three quarters of a cup of chicken salad inside lettuce leaves, fold in the sides, and roll into a cylinder to enjoy.
(Note: The dressing can be refrigerated for up to a week.)

Grilled Filet Steak and Arugula
On those occasions when you want to indulge in some red meat, make it special. Also make sure you include lots of vegetables, especially greens. This is one of my all-time favorites. It's easy and delicious!

Ingredients
Steak
2–4 small filet mignons (If you're only cooking for two, then use only two filet mignons.)
Olive oil, for rubbing
Salt and pepper, to taste

Dressing
1 tablespoon olive oil
½ teaspoon Dijon mustard
2 tablespoons fine sea salt
2 tablespoons coarse black pepper

Salad
4 cups baby arugula

Directions

1. Heat grill (charcoal or gas) to medium heat.
2. Meanwhile, lightly oil and then season filets with salt and pepper.
3. To prepare the dressing, whisk together olive oil, mustard, salt, and pepper and set aside.
4. When grill is ready, cook the steaks for 5 minutes on each side, or until centers are 125 degrees for medium rare, or 7 minutes on each side, until centers are 165 degrees for medium.
5. When steaks are done, set aside and let rest for 5–10 minutes before slicing and plating.
6. Toss arugula with dressing just until leaves are coated (do not saturate) and then scatter over the steaks.

RECOMMENDED STORE-BOUGHT BRANDS

veggie burgers: The Impossible Burger; Praeger's
breakfast sausage: Applegate
frozen pizza: Udi's Cauliflower Pizza

OTHER RESOURCES

Compounding Pharmacies

The list of compounding pharmacies below is provided as a starting point for your research, and more options can be located through the Academy of Anti-Aging Medicine. Always consult with your own trusted medical advisers, who may have more up to date and complete information on any given pharmacy, before choosing a compounding pharmacy.

Tailor Made Compounding
200 Moore Dr.
Nicholasville, KY 40356
859-887-0013
859-406-1242 (fax)
https://tailormadecompounding.com
/contact-us/

Assurance Infusion
2626 South Loop West, Ste. 555
Houston, TX 77054
713-533-8800
1-844-533-8800
713-533-8802
http://assurance.care/

Custom Rx
3510 N. Ridge Rd., Ste. 900
Wichita, KS 67205
316-721-2626
316-721-4823 (fax)
855-287-6879
855-721-4823 (fax)
www.customrx.net/

PD Labs
101 Commercial Parkway
Cedar Park, TX 78613
512-219-0724
512-219-0943 (fax)
www.pdlabs.net/

Sona Compounding Pharmacy
805 Fairview Rd.
Asheville, NC 28803
Pharmacy: 828-298-3636
Clinic: 828-552-3999
https://sonapharmacy.com/contact/

Wells Pharmacy Network
Ocala Pharmacy
1210 SW 33rd Ave.
Ocala, FL 34474

Dyersburg Pharmacy
450 US Highway 51 BYP N.
Dyersburg, TN 38024
www.wellsrx.com/contact/

Finding an Integrative Medical Physician

Academy of Integrative Health and Medicine
www.aihm.org/

Institute for Functional Medicine
www.ifm.org

Bibliography

BENEFITS AND SAFETY OF BIOIDENTICAL ESTROGEN

CARDIOVASCULAR

Compounded transdermal HRT shown to reduce TG, BP, CRP, FIBRINOGEN, GLUCOSE, Factor 7 and significantly improve quality of life. OB GYN news Jan 15 2009. American Heart Association annual meeting. Abstract 5071/poster p-26. Stephenson Kenna.

Estrogen is an ACE-I. Atherosclerosis 2001; 158:391–97. Sanada M et al.

Estrogen increases prostacyclins. Int J Cardiol 2006; 107:19499, Maffei S et al.

Estrogen reduces Endothelin1. Am J Physiol heart cir Physiol 2008; 294:h1630–h1637, Meendering J R et al.

Bioidentical estradiol cream does not increase blood clots or venous thrombosis. Circulation 2007 Feb 20; 115(7): 840–5. Canonico M et al.

Estradiol prevents heart failure. Basic Res Cardiol 2006 Jul 4; Beer S et al.

Bioidentical estradiol protects the heart. Menopause 2006 Jul-Aug; 13(4): 643–50. Zegura B et al.; Basic Res Cardiol 2006 Jul 4; Beer S et al.; Menopause 2001 Jul-Aug: 8(4): 252–8. Ventura P et al.; Ob Gyn News April 15 2005. Wildman RP; Fertil Steril 2004:82:391–7. Mack WJ et al.; Ann NY Acad Sci 1990; 592: 193–203. Stampfer M et al.; Hypertens Res 2005 Jul; 28(7): 579–84. Sumino H et al.

Estrogen decreases erythrocyte deformability. Menopause 2009; 16(3):555–8. Sakashita T.

Low levels of estrogen associated with decrease in vascular tone. Ob Gyn News April 15 2005. Wildman RP.

Low levels of estrogen associated with increase in arterial sclerosis. Fertil Steril 2004:82:391–7. Mack WJ et al.

Low levels of estrogen associated with increased incidence of heart attack and stroke. Ann NY Acad Sci 1990; 592:193–203. Stampfer MJ et al.

Estrogen replacement associated with decrease of 60% in aortal calcification. NEJM 2007 Jun; 356:2591–2602. Manson JE et al.

Estradiol prevents thickening of heart walls. Nucl Recept Signal 2006; 4:e013. Kim JK et al.

Estradiol lowers Homocysteine. Menopause 2001 Jul-Aug: 8(4):252–8. Ventura P et al.

Estradiol decreases the thickening of the carotid artery walls. Hypertens Res 2005 Jul; 28(7):579–84. Sumino H et al.

"The present study demonstrated that estradiol and testosterone have a synergistic effect on early stage atherosclerosis. . . ." Arch Med Res 2015 Nov; 46(8):619–29. Dai W et al.

"Oral estradiol therapy was associated with less progression of subclinical atherosclerosis (measured as CIMT) than was placebo when therapy." N Engl J Med 2016 Mar 31; 374(13):1221–31. Hodis HN et al.

"Women receiving transdermal ET have significantly lower incidences of CVD events compared with those receiving oral ET, and that they also incur lower health care costs." Menopause 2016 Feb 26. Simon JA et al.

"Women who start HRT with E2 within 6 years from menopausal onset show significant slowing of subclinical carotid atherosclerosis, whereas women that are more than 10 years post menopause show no difference from placebo." Menopause 2015; 22(4):391–401. Hodis HN et al.

"The therapeutic benefits of E2 in several pathological events involving endothelial dysfunction and atherosclerosis." Cell Biochem Biophys 2015 Jan 28.

Estradiol improves right ventricular function in rats with severe angioproliferative pulmonary hypertension. Am J Physiol Lung Cell Mol Physiol 2015 May 1; 308(9):L873–90. Frump AL et al.

The discontinuation of HT was accompanied by a significant 33% (1.02–1.72) increase in stroke death risk. Maturitas 2015 Apr 13. pii: S0378-5122(15)00639-8. Tuomikoski P et al.

A total of 40,958 statin users—2,862 (7%) HT users and 38,096 nonusers—were followed for a mean of 4.0 years. Among H(Estradiol progesterone) users, there were five cardiovascular deaths per 10,000 person-years. The corresponding rate among nonusers was 18, which yielded a hazard ratio of 0.38 (68% reduction). Menopause 2015 Apr; 22(4):369–76. Berglind IA et al.

17-β estradiol attenuates ovariectomy-induced changes in cardiomyocyte contractile function. Toxicol Lett 2014 Nov 13; 232(1):253–262. Turdi S et al.

"Study has shown that 17β-estradiol improved myocardial diastolic function, prevented myocardial energy dysregulation, and reduced myocardial oxidative stress in cTnT-Q92 mice." J Steroid Biochem Mol Biol 2015 Mar; 147:92–102. Chen Yet al.

17β-estradiol protects against the progression of hypertension during adulthood in a mouse model of systemic lupus erythematosus. Hypertension 2014 Mar; 63(3):616–623. Gilbert EL et al.

INFLAMMATION

Bioidentical estradiol in cream form decreases inflammation. Gynecol Obstet Mex 2006 Mar; 74(3):133–8. Saucedo Garcia R et al.; Cytokine. 2005 Aug; 31(4):251–7 Liu H et al.

Bioidentical estradiol does not increase CRP. Maturitas 2005 Oct 16; 52(2):111–8. Eilertsen AL et al.; Menopause 2006 Sep-Oct.

Estrogen behaves like an antioxidant. Swiss Med Wkly 2006 Aug 5; 136(31–32):510–4. Delibasi T et al.

Estradiol decreases IL-6. Gynecol Obstet Mex 2006 Mar; 74(3): 133–8. Saucedo Garcia R et al.; J Huazhong Univ Sci Technology Med Sci 2006; 26(1):53–8. Wang Y et al.

Estradiol decreases NFKbeta. Cytokine 2005 Aug 21; 31(4):251–7. Liu H et al.; J Huazhong Univ Sci Technology Med Sci 2006; 26(1):53–8. Wang Y et al.

Estrogen decreases chronic hepatitis fibrosis via antioxidant effect. Braz J Infect Dis 2007 Jun; 11(3):371–4. Codes L et al.

Estrogens control inflammation in experimental colitis. J Biol Regul Homeost Agents 2014 Jul-Sep; 28 2:213–24. Hajj Hussein I et al.

SKIN

Estrogen accelerates wound healing. Endocrinology 2009; 150(6):2749–57. Emerson E et al.

Bioidentical estrogen causes brighter appearance, rounder, fuller, rosier lips. Proc Biol Sci 2006 Jan 22; 273(1583):135–40. Smith MJ et al.

Bioidentical estradiol and estriol cream increases elasticity firmness, decreases wrinkle depth and pore size of the skin. Int J Dermatology 1996 Sep; 35(9):669–74. Schmidt JB et al.; Climacteric 2007 Aug; 10(4):289–97. Verdier-Sevrain S.

The postmenopausal decrease in estrogen circulating levels results in rapid skin deterioration pointing out to a protective effect exerted by these hormones. PLoS One 2015 Mar 17; 10(3):e0120672. Carnesecchi J et al.

Prophylactic BSO during hysterectomy is a significant independent risk factor for worsening skin laxity/sagging and texture/dryness in premenopausal women undergoing hysterectomy for benign conditions. Menopause 2016 Feb; 23(2):138–42. Töz E et al.

Vaginal estrogen application for 6 weeks preoperatively increased synthesis of mature collagen, decreased degradative enzyme activity, and increased thickness of the vaginal wall. J Clinic Endocrinol Metab 2014 Jun. Rahn DD et al.

AUTOIMMUNE AND BRAIN

Bioidentical HRT protection from Parkinson. JAMA Neurol. 2018 Mar 1: 75(3): 312–319. Saunders-Pullman R et al.

E2 and DHT improve RA in experimental mice. Calcif Tissue Int 2008 Nov; 83(5):354–364. Ganesan K et al.

Estrogen protective to the liver from the severity of fibrosis. Hepatology 2013 Oct 1. Yang JD et al.

Pregnancy level of estrogen attenuates experimental autoimmune encephalomyelitis. J Neuroimmunol 2014 Dec 15; 277(1-2):85–95. Haghmorad D et al.

Failing to maintain estrogen levels may cause permanent memory loss. J Neuro Endocrinol 2007 Feb; 19(2):77–81. Sherwin BB.

A 3-day estrogen treatment improves prefrontal cortex–dependent cognitive function in postmenopausal women. Psychoneuroendocrinology 2006 Sep; 31(8):965–75. Krug R et al.

"Add-back" estrogen reverses cognitive deficits induced by a gonadotropin-releasing hormone agonist in women with leiomyoma uteri. J Clinic Endo Meta. 81:2545–2549. Sherwin BB et al.

Estrogen improves levels of acetylcholine. Brain Res 2000; 864(2):263–69. Farr SA et al.

Estradiol interacts with the cholinergic system to affect verbal memory in postmenopausal women: Evidence for the critical period hypothesis. Horm Behav 2008 Jan; 53(1):159–169. Dumas J et al.

Estrogen improves levels of serotonin. Psychopharmacology Bull 1997; 33(2):229–33. Chakravorty SG et al.

Estrogen enhances norepinephrine function. Endocrinology 2002 Oct; 143(10):3974–83. Temel S et al.

Estrogen increases executive function and cognitive function. Horm Behav 2006 Dec 13. Norbury R et al.

Estrogen increases verbal memory. Ann NY Acad Sci 2005 Jun; 1052:3–10. Sherwin BB.

Estrogen increases cognitive recognition: Women Health 2006; 43(1):37–57. Stephens C et al.

Estrogen increases spatial memory. Neurobiology Aging 2006 Apr 16. Harburger LL et al.

Estrogen protects against injury from stroke. Trends Neurosci 2001 Jul; 24(7):386–91. Stein DG.

Estrogen protects against injury from epilepsy. Neuroscientist 2007 Feb; 13(1):77–88. Veliskova J.

Estrogen increases BDNF. Front Neuro Endocrinol 2006 Oct 19; Scharfman HE et al.

Estrogen prevents brain grey matter loss. Menopause 2006 Jul-Aug; 13(4):584–91. Bacardi M et al.

Estrogen prevents brain white matter loss. Neurobiology Aging 2006 Oct 6. Ha DM et al.

Estrogen protects against Alzheimer's disease. Adv Etp Meg Bio. 1997; 429:261–71. Chang D et al.; Menopause 2006 Jul-Aug; 13(4):584–91. Boccardi M et al. Neurology. 57:605–612. Asthana S et al.; Proc Natl Acad Sci USA. 2005.102:19198–19203.

Estrogen protects against stress-induced damage to hippocampus cells. Neuroscience 2007 Feb 21. Takuma K et al.

Estrogen treatment improves visual function. Menopause 2003; 10(1)53. Guaschimo S et al.

Estradiol slightly decreases cataract formation. Int Ophthalmology 2009 Dec 5. Ozcura F et al.

Estrogen treatment prevents intraocular pressure and improves amount/quality of eye lubrication. Ophthalmologica 2004 Mar-Apr; 218(2):120–9. Altintas O et al.

Estrogen regulates functions of RPE (Retinal Pigment Epithelium) and its deficiency during menopause period may be a factor contributing to the development of age-related macular degeneration in elderly women. Mech Ageing Dev 2005 Nov; 126(11):1135–45.Yu X et al.

Estrogen deficiency is associated with age-related hearing loss. Amer J Ob/Gyn 2004 Jan; 190(1):77–82. Kilicdag EB et al.

Low-dose estradiol patch provides too little to benefit cognitive function. Arch Neurol 2006 Jul; 63(7):945–50. Yaffe K et al.

Intermittent dosing of estrogen impairs cognition. Brain Res 2006 Oct 18; 1115(1):135–47. Gresack JE et al.

Duration of estrogen deprivation, not chronological age, prevents estrogen's ability to enhance hippocampal synaptic physiology. Proc Natl Acad Sci USA. 2010 Nov; 107 (45):1543–8. Smith CC et al.

"role of neurosteroids especially that of oestrogen in AD . . . maintenance and function of mitochondria." Mol Neurol 2012 Jun.* Grimm A.

17β-estradiol mediated rapid formation of new dendritic spines in the hippocampus. Neuropsychopharmacol 2012 Jun 6. Phan A et al.

Estradiol attenuates spinal cord injury–related central pain by decreasing glutamate levels in thalamic VPL nucleus in male rats. Meta Brain Dis 2014 May 31. Naderi A et al.

Estradiol is neuroprotective, promotes synaptic plasticity in the hippocampus, and protects against cognitive decline associated with aging and neurodegenerative diseases. J Neurosci 2015 Dec 9; 35(49):16077–93. Bean LA et al.

High-dose estrogen treatment at reperfusion reduces lesion volume and accelerates recovery of sensorimotor function after experimental ischemic stroke. Brain Res 2016 Mar 1. Carpenter RS et al.

Treatment with ovarian hormones can partially improve spatial learning and memory deficits induced by methamphetamine in OVX rats. Neurosci Lett 2016 Apr 21; 619:60–7. Ghazvini H et al.

Neuroprotective effects of estrogen and progesterone after traumatic brain injury (TBI) and spinal cord injury. Curr Neuropharmacol 2016 Mar 9. Brotfain et al.

"Results showed that long-term 17β-estradiol treatment has positive effects on both reference memory and working memory and that ACh vesicles increased in the examined brain areas, especially in hippocampus." 2016 Feb 15. Uzum G et al.

The neuroprotective effect of 17β-estradiol is independent of its antioxidative properties. Brain Res 2014 Aug 20; 1589C:61–67. Gröger M and Plesnila N.

BONE AND MUSCLE

Bioidentical estradiol promotes muscle growth and regeneration. J Appl Physiol 2006 Jun; 100(6):2012–23. McClung JM et al.

Significant increase of osteoporosis and bone fracture when women stop taking estrogen. Climacteric 2007 Aug; 10(4):273–5. Gambaccini M et al.

Estrogen is also important for maintaining bone formation at the cellular level. Trend Endocrinol Meta 2012 May 15. Khosla S et al.

Estrogen is a crucial hormone for osteoclast inhibition and for preventing osteoporosis. J Cell Biochem 2015 Jul; 116(7):1419–30. Wu SM et al.

Declines in endogenous estrogen levels after menopause can lead to systemic bone loss, including loss of oral bone. J Periodontol 2015 Apr; 86(4):595–605. Wang Y et al.

Oestrogen deficiency causes maxillary alveolar bone loss. Arch Oral Biol 2015 Feb; 60(2):333–41. Macari S et al.

Skeletal muscle action of estrogen receptor α is critical for the maintenance of mitochondrial function and metabolic homeostasis in females. Transl Med 2016 Apr 13; 8(334):334ra54. Ribas V et al.

MOOD

Postpartum estrogen withdrawal impairs hippocampal neurogenesis and causes depression- and anxiety-like behaviors. Psychoneuroendocrinology 2016 Apr; 66:138–49. Zhang Z et al.

Produced 238 patients whose principal presenting symptom was depression, given estradiol and progesterone. For 94%, the hormone therapy was a life-changing event for the better. None were worse. Post Reprod Health 2014 Dec; 20(4):132–7. Studd J.

Meaningful elevations in depressive symptoms increase two- to threefold during the menopause transition. Am J Psychiatry 2015 Mar 1; 172(3):227–36. Gordon JL et al.

Estrogen is protective in schizophrenia. Psychopharmacology 2012 Jan 219(1):213–24. Gagos A et al.

Estradiol decreases cortisol. Neuro Endocrinol Lett 2006 Oct; 27(5)659–64. Kerdelhue B et al.

Bioidentical estrogen has a significant positive effect on panic attacks. Orv Hetil 2006 May 14; 147(19):879–85. Magyar Z et al.

Estrogen increases serotonin. Biol Psychiatry 2000; 47(6):562–576. Bethea CL et al.

Low levels of estrogen in beginning of woman's cycle are associated with depression. Arch Gen Psychiatry 2000 Dec; 57(12):1157–62. Young EA et al.

Women in perimenopause experience greater incidence of depression. North American Menopause Society 2007. Schmidt PJ et al.

Depressed women enter menopause earlier. Arch Gen Psychiatry 2001 June; 58(6):529-34. Soares CN et al.

Estrogen improves mood, decreases postpartum depression and anxiety. Psychoneuroendocrinology 2007 May; 32(4):350–7. Hill MN, Karacabeyli ES, Gorzalka BB.

Postpartum depression and psychosis successfully treated with estrogen. J Clin Psychiatry 2000 Mar; 61(3):166–9. Ahokcas A et al.

Nonresponsive depression successfully treated with estradiol. Arch Gen Psychiatry 1997 May; 36(5):550–4. Klaiber EL et al.

Depressed perimenopausal women who do not respond to SSRI after administration of estrogen improve their mood. J Clin Psychiatry 2002; 63 Suppl 7:45–8. Rasgon NL et al.

Estrogen acts as an MAO inhibitor. Psychopharmacology Bull 1997; 33(2):229–33. Chakravorty SG et al.

ESTROGEN PROTECTS AGAINST MIGRAINE

Migraines are more frequent on days estrogen levels decline. Headache 2006 Oct; 46 Suppl 2:S49–54. Zacur HA.

Migraines more frequent immediately after delivery. Neurology 1972; 22:355. Somerville et al.

Menstrual migraines are due to low level of estrogen. Neurology 1991 Jun; 41(6):786–93. Silberstein SD et al.

17β-estradiol but not estriol plays an antihyperalgesic role in physiological pain. Steroid 2012 Feb; 77(3)):241–9. Lu Y et al.

"17β-estradiol can exert protective effect on decrease of inflammation in migraine." Iran J Basic Med Sci 2015 Sep; 18(9)894–901 Karkhaneh A et al.

METABOLISM AND WEIGHT LOSS, MITOCHONDRIA AND DIABETES

Estrogen controls mitochondrial function and biogenesis. Cell Biochem 2008 Dec; 105(6):1342–51. Kline CM.

In the ovariectomized female rats model, exogenous estrogen can significantly up-regulate telomerase activity and TERT mRNA expression to exert the effects of anti-aging. Gynecol Endocrinol 2015 Jul; 31(7):582–5. Cen J et al.

E2 promotes the energetic capacity of brain mitochondria by maximizing aerobic glycolysis (preventing AD). Adv Drug Deliv Rev 2008 Oct-Nov; 30(13-14): 1504–11. Brinton RD et al.

Estrogen prevents cell death by maintaining functionally intact mitochondria. Brain Res Rev 2008 Mar; 57(2):421–30. Simpkins JW et al.

HRT treatment in postmenopausal women decreases the incidence of diabetes. Eur J Endocrinol 2009 Jun; 160(6):979–983. Pentti K et al.

Bioidentical estradiol decreases body fat. Philos Trans R Soc Lond B Biol Sci 2006 Jul 29; 361(1471):1251–63. Asarian L et al.

Bioidentical estradiol applied to skin decreases ghrelin. Fertil Steril 2006 Dec; 86(6)1669. Micheline CC et al.

Bioidentical estradiol increases CCK, satiety, and decreases food intake. Philos Trans R Soc Lond B Biol Sci 2006 Jul 29; 361(1471):1251–63. Asarian L et al.

Decline of estrogen leads to binge-eating. Psychol Med 2006 Oct 12:1–11. Edler C et al.

Prolonged estradiol treatment increases insulin sensitivity. Mol Endocrinol 2006 Jun; 20(6):1287–99. Gao H et al.

Bioidentical estradiol cream is more effective in managing weight and insulin sensitivity than capsule form. Fertil Steril 2006 Dec; 86(6)1669. Micheline CC et al.

Estradiol helps overcome leptin resistance in mice on high-fat diet. Horm Metab Res 2010 Mar; 42(3):182–6. Matyskova R et al.

Prevention of obesity and insulin resistance by estrogens. Diabetes 2013; July 31. Handgraaf S et al.

Duration of estrogen deficiency in postmenopausal state confers fibrosis risk among postmenopausal women with NAFLD. Hepatology 2016 Feb 26. Klair JS et al.

GENERAL HEALTH BENEFITS OF BIOIDENTICAL HORMONES

Estradiol as positive treatment for postpartum depression. J Clin Psychopharmacol 2015 Aug; 35(4):389–95. Wisner KL et al.

The association between vulvar pain and bladder pain is related to a vaginal environment carrying signs of hypoestrogenism. Gynecol Endocrinol 2015 Oct; 31(10):828–32. Gardella B et al.

Hormone replacement, as reported here, could possibly slow the loss of alveoli due to the aging process. Anat Rec (Hoboken) 2016 Apr 16. Herring MJ et al.

New-onset asthma and respiratory symptoms increased in women becoming postmenopausal. Allergy Clin Immunol 2016 Jan; 137(1):50–57e6. Triebner K et al.

Estriol acting through ER alpha to reduce MMP-9 from immune cells is one mechanism potentially underlying the estriol-mediated reduction in enhancing lesions in MS and inflammatory lesions in EAE (experimental autoimmune encephalomyelitis). Lab Invest 2009 Oct; 89(10):1076–83. Gold SM et al.

Estriol treatment in multiple sclerosis. Prog Brain Res 2009; 175:239–51. Gold SM et al.

Estriol restores vaginal integrity. Menopause 2009 Sep-Oct; 16(5):978–83. Chollet JA et al.

Protective effects of estriol established more than thirty-five years ago. Ann Intern Med 1978 Sep; 89(3):422–3. Lemon HM.

Estriol does not promote uterine tissue growth, which may decrease the incidence of uterine cancer. Comp Biochem Physiol C 1990; 96(2):241–4. Tamaya T et al.; JAMA 1978 Apr 21; 239(16):1638–41. Tzingounis VA et al.

Estriol quickly alleviates night sweats and hot flashes: JAMA 1978 Apr 21; 239(16):1638–41. Tzingounis VA et al.; Zhonghua Yi Xue Za Zhi (Taipei) 1995 May; 55(5):386–91. Yang TS et al.; Maturitas 2000 Feb 15; 34(2):169–77. Takahashi K et al.

Estriol decreases NFKbeta. J TNF-alpha Neuroimmunol 2002 Mar; 124(1-2): 106–14. Zang YC et al.

Estriol reduces coronary hyperactivity. Am J Physiol Heart Circ Physiol 2006 Jan; 290(1): H 295–303. Mishra RG et al.

Estriol may help build bone. Gynecol Endocrinol 2003 Dec; 17(6):455–61. Yamanaka Y et al.

UCLA study of bioidentical estriol in the treatment of MS. Neurology 1999 Apr 12; 52(6):1230–8. Kim S et al.; J Immunol 2003 Dec 1; 171(11):6267–74. Soldan SS et al.; Ann Neurol 2002 Oct; 52(4):421–8. Sicotte NL et al.

Estrogen beta receptor deficiency may cause interstitial cystitis. Proc Natl Acad Sci USA. 2007 Jun 5; 104(23):9806–9. Imamov O et al.; J Endocrinol 2007 June; 193(3):421–33. Treeck O et al.

Estriol affects beta receptors that decrease breast tissue proliferation. Endocrinology 2006 Sep; 147(9):4132–50. Zhu BT et al.; Endocrinology 2007; 148(2):538–547. Cvoro A et al.

Estriol prevents breast cancer cells from producing new blood vessels and VEGF. Cancer Res 2006 Dec 1; 66(23):11207–13. Hartman J et al.

Estriol has anti-tumor effect on ovarian cancer cell. J Endocrinol 2007 Jun; 19 Beta estrogen receptor knockout (BERKO) mice show profound memory impairment in a hippocampus-mediated fear-conditioning paradigm. Behav Brain Res 2005 Oct; 164(1):128–131. Day et al.

E(2)'s anti-anxiety and antidepressive effects may involve ERbeta in the hippocampus. Pharmacol Biochem Behav 2007 Feb; 86(2):407–14. Epub 2006 Aug 17. Walf AA et al.

Estriol, an estrogen, at 0.6nmol/l was reported to inhibit platelet aggregation. Blood Coagulation Fibrinolysis 2014 Apr. Jana P et al.

"Estriol short-term therapy modulates within 10 days of administration the neuro-endocrine control of the hypothalamus-pituitary unit and induces the recovery of both gonadotropin synthesis and secretion in hypogonadotropic patients with FHA (Functional Hypothalamic Amenorhea)." Gynecol Endocrinol 2016 Mar; 32(3):253–7. Genazzani AD et al.

Stage I and II Stress Incontinence (SIC): High dosed vitamin D may improve effects of local estriol. Dermatoendocrinol 2016 Apr 19; 8(1):e1079359. Schulte-Uebbing C et al.

For children <5 years of age a 4-week topical therapy with estriol is a promising therapy option for synechia of the labia that is less of a burden for the family situation (80% success rate). Geburtshilfe Frauenheilk 2016 Apr; 76(4):390–395. Bussen S et al.

Application of topical estriol ointment is an effective treatment for hereditary hemorrhagic telangiectasia (HHT) epistaxis. Acta Otolaryngol 2016 May; 136(5):528–31. Minami K et al.

BENEFITS OF BIOIDENTICAL PROGESTERONE

Bioidentical progesterone decreases apoptosis. Biol Reprod 2004 Dec; 71(6):2065–71. Okuda K et al.

Balancing effect of estrogen by progesterone important for preventing development of cancer. J Clin Endo Metab 2002; 87(1):3–15. Hale et al.; Proc Natl Acad Sci USA 2006 Sep 19; 103(38):14021–6. Pan H et al.

Anti-tumor effects of progesterone in human glioblastoma multiforme. J Steroid Biochem Mol Biol 2014 Apr. Atif F et al.

Progesterone significantly inhibited mouse melanoma cell growth in vitro, progesterone inhibited human melanoma cell growth also in vitro. The mechanism of inhibition was due to autophagy and this effect of progesterone was not mediated through progesterone receptor. Int J Clin Exp Med 2014 Nov 15; 7(11):3941–53. eCollection 2014. Ramaraj P and Cox JL.

Higher level of progesterone during pregnancy associated with 80 percent decrease in breast cancer. Cancer Epi Bio Prev April 2002; 11(4):381–8. Peck JD et al.

Use of estradiol and progesterone in menopause is not associated with increase in breast cancer in difference to chemical HRT that does increase breast cancer risk if given in menopause. J Clin Oncol 2009 Nov; 27(31):5116–9. Fournier A et al.

E2 in high level in the presence of progesterone, upregulate ER-beta receptors and down regulate E2-alpha receptors. J Clin Endo Meta 2005; 90(1):435–444. Cheng G et al.

Bioidentical progesterone does not increase breast cancer; progestin does increase breast cancer. Steroid Biochem Mol Biol 2005 July; 96(2):95–108. Campagnoli C et al.

Progesterone blocks NFk-Beta and Cox-2 and protects breast cancer. J Steroid Biochem Mol Biol 2006 Oct 16. Mendelson CR et al.

Progesterone protects breast tissue from HER 2/new oncogenic. J Steroid Biochem Mol Biol 2006 Dec; 102(1-5):241–9. Mendelson CR et al.

Perioperative progesterone for obese women with breast cancer may improve survival. Women's Health (London England) 2016 Mar; 12(2):179–84. Fentiman IS.

Bioidentical progesterone protects from breast cancer. Proc Natl Acad Sci USA 2003 Sep 2; 100(18):10506–11. Nielsen J; J Steroid Biochem Mol Biol 2001 Aug; 78(2):185–91. McDonnell AC et al.; Clin Cancer Res 2001 Sep; 7(9):2880–6. Lin VC et al.; Am J Epidemiol 1981; 114(2):209–17. Cowan LD; Int J Cancer 2005 Apr 10; 114(3):448–54. Fournier A; Pathol Biol 1987; 35:1081–86. Mauvais-Jarvis P; Ann NY Acad Sci 1986; 464:152–67. Mauvais-Jarvis P; Cancer Detect Prev 1999; 23:290–298. Plu-Bureau G; Climacteric 2002; 5:332–40. Lignieres

B; Breast Cancer Res Treat 2006 Jul 14. Wood CE. J Steroid Biochem Mol Biol 2006 Oct 16. Mendelson CR; Breast J 2006 Nov; 12(6):518–525. Kontos M; J Steroid Biochem Mol Biol 2006 Dec; 102(1-5):241–9. Mendelson CR et al.

P4 (progesterone) exposure of cells resulted in increased p-53 and BAX and decreased BCL-2 expression. Gynecol Endocrin 2010 Dec 21. Nguyen H et al.

Progesterone inhibits growth and induces apoptosis in breast cancer cells: inverse effects on Bcl-2. Annals of Clinic and Lab Science 1998: 28(6):360–369. Formby B et al.

Micronized progesterone does not increase cell proliferation in breast tissue in postmenopausal women. Climacteric 2012 Apr; 15 Supp1:18–25. Gompel.

The administration of 200 mg/day progesterone over 12 days of a menstrual cycle or a daily administration of 100 mg combined with an estrogen are a safe and well-tolerated option to treat menopausal symptoms, with a better benefit risk profile compared to synthetic gestagens. Geburtshilfe Frauenheilk 2014 Nov; 74(11):995–1002. Regidor PA.

Loss of PR expression in primary tumors is associated with a less differentiated more invasive phenotype and worse prognosis, suggesting that PR may limit later stages of tumor progression. Mol Cell Endocrinol 2012 Jun 24; 357(1-2): 4–17. Obr AE et al.

High Ki-67 Expression and Low Progesterone Receptor Expression Could Independently Lead to a Worse Prognosis for Postmenopausal Patients with Estrogen Receptor-Positive and HER2-Negative Breast Cancer. Clin Breast Cancer 2014 Dec 24. Nishimukai A et al.

Johns Hopkins study indicates significant increase in mortality, cancer, and breast cancer in women who had low progesterone versus normal progesterone. Am J Epidemiol 1981; 114(2):209–17. Cowan LD et al.

Mice given high doses of estrogen and progesterone at puberty reduced breast cancer by 60 percent and eliminated HER-2/neu (HER-2). Breast Cancer Res 2007 Jan 26; 9(1): R12. Rajkumar L et al.

"Around half of all breast cancer patients could one day benefit from having the cheap and widely available female hormone progesterone added to their treatment, according to Cancer Research UK-funded research published in Nature (link is external). Women whose tumours have progesterone receptors as well are known to have a better outlook. Scientists at Cancer Research UK's Cambridge Research Institute (link is external) and the University of Adelaide (link is external) revealed how the progesterone receptor 'talks to' the oestrogen receptor in breast cancer cells to change their behaviour, ultimately slowing down tumour growth." Nature 2015 July; 523(7560):313–7. Carroll J et al.

Progesterone elicited an increase in BNDF and decreased glutamate toxicity. J Neurosci Res 2007 Aug 15; 85(11):2441–9. Kaur P et al.

Bioidentical progesterone protects neurological system. J Neurobiol 2006 Aug; 66(9):916–28. Ciriza I et al.; Endocrine 2006 Apr; 29(2):271–4. Singh M.

Bioidentical progesterone increases GABA and Allopregnenolone and is a brain calmer. J Neuro Endocrinol 1995 Mar; 7(3):171–7. Bitrn D; Brain Res 1995 May 22; 680(1-2):135–41. Picazo O et al.

Bioidentical progesterone improves memory by calming, improving sleep, and providing general cognitive protection. Ann NY Acad Sci 2005 Jun; 1052:152–69. Stein DG.

Progesterone increases myelin. J Neurotrauma 2006 Feb; 23(2):181–92. Labombarda F et al.

Progesterone significantly aids in decreasing brain edema. Pharmacol Biochem Behav 2006 Jul; 84(3):420–8. Cutler SM et al.

Progesterone shown to prevent damage caused by brain trauma and to enhance the rate of recovery. Neuroscience 2004; 123(2):349–59. Djebaili M et al.; Exp Neurol 2002 Nov; 178(1):59–67. Shear DA et al.

Progesterone decreases mortality of brain trauma by more than 50%, improves and accelerates recovery. Ann Emer Med 2008 Feb; 51(12):164–72. Stein DG et al.

Women given chemicalized progesterone for five years and switched to bioidentical progesterone for 6 months improved mood, decreased anxiety and depression. J Women's Health Gend Base Med 2000 May; 9(4):381–7. Fitzpatrick LA et al.

Progesterone improves hearing. Neuropsychologia 2002; 40(8):1293–9. Alexander GM et al.

Progesterone protects from seizures. J Neuro Endocrinol 1995 Mar; 7(3):171–7. Bitran D et al.; Brain Res 1995 May 22; 680(1-2):135–41. Picazo O et al.

Progesterone decreases cocaine craving. Exp Clin Psychopharmaco 2007 Oct; 15(5):472–80. Anker JJ et al.

Progesterone and allopregnenolone attenuate blood-brain barrier dysfunction following permanent focal ischemia by regulating the expression of matrix metalloproteinase. Exp Neurol 2010 Sep 15. Ishrat T et al.

Progesterone protects hippocampal cultures from cell death. Neuroscience Lett 2016; 506(1):131–5. Radley E et al.

Progesterone effectively protects the spinal cord tissues against ischemic damage in the setting of decreased perfusion. AM J Emerg Med 2012 Nov 16. Kara PH et al.

Progesterone treatment reduces neuroinflammation, oxidative stress and brain damage and improves long-term outcomes in a rat model of repeated mild traumatic brain injury. J Neuroinflammation 2015 Dec 18; 12:238. Webster KM et al.

"treatment with ovarian hormones can partially improve spatial learning and memory deficits induced by methamphetamine in OVX rats." Neurosci Lett 2016 Apr 21; 619:60–7. Ghazvini H et al.

Progesterone protects mitochondrial function in a rat model of pediatric traumatic brain injury. J Bioenerg Biomembr 2015 Apr; 47(1-2):43–51. Robertson CL et al.

Identical progesterone promotes better sleep. Poster Endocrinology Conference 2004 New Orleans. Callfries A; Menopause 2001; 8(1):10–16. Montplaisir J et al.; Curr Med Chem 2006; 13(29):3575–82. Andersen ML et al.

"We tested the hypothesis that the nuclear progesterone receptor (nPR) is involved in respiratory control and mediates the respiratory stimulant effect of progesterone. We conclude that the nPR reduces apnea frequency during non-REM sleep and enhances chemoreflex responses to hypercapnia after progesterone treatment." PLoS One 2014 Jun 19; 9(6):e100421. Marcouiller F et al.

Bioidentical progesterone decreases mast cells. Int J Immunopathol Pharmacol 2006 Oct-Dec; 19(4):787–94. Vasiadi M et al.

Progesterone improves immunity. J Cell Biochem 2006 Sep 1; 99(1):292–304. Chien EJ et al.

Progesterone decreases allergies. Int J Immunopathol Pharmacol 2006 Oct-Dec; 19(4):787–94. Vasiadi M et al.

Progesterone decreases interstitial cystitis and IBS. Int J Immunopathol Pharmacol 2006 Oct-Dec; 19(4):787–94. Vasiadi M et al.

Progesterone Protective Effects in Neurodegeneration and Neuroinflammation. J Neuroendocrinology 2013 May. De Nicola AF et al.

Natural progesterone is effective against endometriosis in rat model. Clin Exp Obstst Gynecol 2014; 41(4):455–9. Narin R et al.

Foci of endometriosis proliferate under estrogen stimulation, like normal endometrium . . . under progesterone hormonal replacement and cessation of estradiol. Clin Nucl Med 2016 Mar; 41(3):e143–5. Arsenault F et al.

Progesterone significantly enhances fertility. J Clinic Endo Meta 1987; 64:865–7. Brzezinski A et al; Fertil Steril 2003; 80:1012–6. Nakamura Y et al.

Progesterone reduces fibroid formation. Steroids 2000; 65:585–592. Matsuo MT et al.

Progesterone improves cardiovascular function. J Clin Endo Meta 2000; 85:4644–4649. Mather KJ et al.

Bioidentical progesterone does not promote diabetes. Euro J Endo 1999; 140(3):215–223. Cucinelli F et al.; Exp Physiol 2007 Jan; 92(1):241–9. Ordonez et al.

Bioidentical progesterone decreases water retention. Horm Metab Res 2004 Jun; 36(6):381–6. Quinkler M et al.

Patients treated with vaginal progesterone gel (Crinone 90 mg) twice daily had a lower risk of pregnancy loss (43.7%). Repro Biomed Online 2013 Feb; 26(2):133–7. Alsbjerg B et al.

Bioidentical progesterone builds bone. Endocr Res 2003 Nov; 29(4):483–501. Liang M et al.; Di Yi Jun Yi Da Xue Xue Bao 2001; 21(12):929–931. Zhang P et al.; Calcif Tissue Int 2002 Oct; 71(4):329–34. Luo XH et al.; J Tongji Med Univ. 2000; 20(1):59–62. Chen L et al.

P(4) prevents bone loss in pre- and possibly perimenopausal women; progesterone cotherapy with antiresorptives may increase bone formation and BMD. J Osteoporosis 2010 Oct; 2010:845180. Prior JC et al.

Progesterone therapy in women with intractable catamenial epilepsy. Adv Biomed Res 2013 Mar; 2:8. Najafi M et al.

Findings support AP (allopregnenolone) as a mediator of seizure reduction in progesterone-treated women with epilepsy. Neurology 2014 Jul 22; 83(4):345–8. Herzog AG and Frye CA.

Pregnancy normalized familial hyperaldosteronism type I: A novel role for progesterone. J Hum Hypertension 2014 Jun. Campino C et al.

Progesterone may have a potential benefit in treatment of benign prostatic hypertrophy (BPH), prostate cancer. J Pharma Pharmacol 012Aug; 64(8):1040–62. Kaore SN et al.

SIGNIFICANT RESEARCH ON HORMONAL HEALTH AND OTHER CONDITIONS

INSOMNIA

Sleep disturbance in menopause. Intern Med J 2012 Jul; 42(7):742–7. Ameratunga D et al.

Study suggests that women who routinely sleep fewer hours may develop more aggressive breast cancers compared with women who sleep longer hours. Breast Cancer Research Treatment 2012 134(3):1291–1295. Li Li et al.

Better sleep efficiency was found to predict a significant reduction in overall mortality (by 4%). Sleep 2014 May 37(5):837–42. Palesh O et al.

Hypnotics association with mortality or cancer: A matched cohort study. Receiving hypnotic prescriptions was associated with greater than threefold increased hazards of death even when prescribed <18 pills a year. Hypnotic use in the upper third was associated with a significant elevation of incident cancer; HR=1.35 (95% CI 1.18 to 1.55). Results were robust within groups suffering each comorbidity, indicating that the death and cancer hazards associated with hypnotic drugs were not attributable to pre-existing disease. BMJ Open 2012 Feb 27; 2(1):e000850. Kripke DF et al.

Restless sleep has been associated with triple negative BC (breast cancer) increase, by 250%. Sleep less than 6 hours, this association with BC increases by 25%. Breast Cancer Res Treat 2017 Jul; 164(1):169–178. Hale L et al.

Frequent waking during the night is associated with increase of BC by 21%. European J Cancer Prev 2018 .10.1097/CEJ. Yang W et al.

This nationwide population-based cohort study reveals that insomnia but not hypnotic use of meds is associated with an increased risk of breast cancer by 43%. J Women's Health (Larchmt) 2018 Mar 12. Chiu HY et al.

ANXIETY AND STRESS

Stress increases risk of breast cancer. Am J Epidemiol 2003 Mar 1; 157(5):415–23. Lillberg K et al.

Significant stress doubles breast cancer risk. LA Times 2002 Sep 24; Med Hypotheses 2007; 68(5):1138–43. Gago-Dominguez M et al.; Mol Cell Biochem 2007 Aug 11. Zweitzig DR et al.

Stress increases metastasis and circulating tumor cell in breast cancer. Mol Cell Biochem 2007 Dec; 306(1-2):255–60. Zweitzig DR et al.

Stress history increases recurrence of breast cancer. J Psychosomatic Res 2007 Sep; 63(3):233–9. Palesh O et al.

Menopause increases depression by 46%. BMC Women's Health 2017 Dec 8; 17(1):124. Yisna E et al.

"We observed a moderate, although significant, reduction in markers of the stress-response to mental arithmetic in postmenopausal women treated with transdermal 17-beta-estradiol." Am J Med 2000 Oct 15; 109(6):463–8. Ceresini G et al.

Chronic stress increases BC metastasis. Psychoneuroendocrinology 2018 Sep 15; 99:191–195. Walker AK et al.

DEPRESSION

Depression as a predictor of disease progression and mortality in cancer patients. Cancer 2009 115(22):5349–61. Satin JR et al.

Major depression was associated with significant increased risk of breast cancer — 380%. Cancer Causes Control 2000 Sep; 11(8):751–8. Gallo JJ et al.

Estrogen acts as an MAO Inhibitor. Psychopharmacology Bull 1997; 33(2):229–33. Chakravorty SG et al.

Estrogen improves production of serotonin and norepinephrine. Brain Res 2000; 864(2):263–69. Farr SA et al.

Nonresponsive depression successfully treated with estradiol. Arch Gen Psychiatry 1997 May; 36(5):550–4. Klaiber EL et al.

Depressed perimenopausal women who do not respond to SSRI after administration of estrogen improve their mood. J Clin Psychiatry 2002; 63 Suppl 7:45–8. Rasgon NL et al.

"SSRIs may elevate risks of ER+/PR- tumors." Breast Cancer Res Treat 2006 Jan; 95(2):131–40. Chien C et al.

Paroxetine use was associated with an increase in breast cancer risk. Am J Epidemiology 2000 May; 151(10):951–7. Cotterchio M et al.

Breast cancer patients on tamoxifen that were given Paroxetine increased their death by up to 91%. BMJ 2010 Feb 8; 340:c693. Kelly CM et al.

SSRI use overall increased death by over 30% in menopausal women and 45% increase of stroke, 220% increase in hemorrhagic stroke, and 210% in fatal stroke. Arch Inte Med 2009 Dec; 169(22):2128–39. Smoller JW et al.

Treatment with SSRI and TCA (tricyclic) might be associated with increased lung cancer risk (27%). SSRI therapy might be associated with modest increase in breast cancer risk (12%). Eur Neuropsychopharmacol 2015 Aug; 25(8):1147–57. Boursi B et al.

CARDIOVASCULAR DECLINE

Bioidentical estradiol protects the heart. Menopause 2006 Jul-Aug; 13(4):643–50. Zegura B et al.; Basic Res Cardiol 2006 Jul 4; Beer S et al.; Menopause 2001 Jul-Aug: 8(4):252–8. Ventura P et al.; Ob Gyn News Apr 15 2005. Wildman RP; Fertil Steril 2004:82:391–7. Mack WJ et al.; Hypertens Res 2005 Jul; 28(7):579–84. Sumino H et al.

The cardiac and stroke death risk elevations were even higher when compared to HT users. Clin Endocrinol Metab 2015 Sep 28:100(12): 4588–94. Mikkola TS et al.

The discontinuation of HT was accompanied by a significant increase in stroke death risk. Maturitas 2015 Apr 13. pii: S0378–5122(15)00639-8. Tuomikoski P et al.

A total of 40,958 statin users—2,862 (7%) HT users and 38,096 nonusers—were followed for a mean of 4.0 years. Among H (Estradiol progesterone) users, there were five cardiovascular deaths per 10,000 person-years. The corresponding rate among nonusers was 18, which yielded a hazard ratio of 0.38 (68% reduction. Menopause 2015 Apr; 22(4):369–76. Berglind IA et al.

Low levels of estrogen associated with increased incidence of heart attack and stroke. Ann NY Acad Sci 1990; 592:193–203. Stampfer MJ et al.

The response of the adaptive immune system to ovarian hormone deficiency is a significant contributor to hypertension in women. Exp Physiol 2015 Sep 30. Sandberg K et al.

New cardiac benefit of menopausal hormonal therapy. Climacteric 2017 Jan; 2:1–6; Mikkola TS et al.

Protective effects of estrogen against vascular calcification via estrogen receptor α-dependent growth arrest specific gene 6 transactivation. Potential therapeutic strategy for the prevention of vascular calcification, especially in postmenopausal women. Biochem Biophys Res Commun 2016 Nov 18; 480(3):429–435. Nanao-Hamai M et al.

Sex steroids have profound effects on many CHD (coronary heart disease) risk factors. Curr Vasc Pharmacol 2018 Oct 2. Stevenson JC et al.

CENTRAL NERVOUS SYSTEM AND THE BRAIN

Bioidentical HRT protects from Parkinson. Saunders-Pullman R neurology meeting 2009.

Failing to maintain estrogen levels may cause permanent memory loss. J Neuro Endocrinol 2007 Feb; 19(2):77–81. Sherwin BB.

Estrogen protects against injury from stroke. Trends Neurosci 2001 Jul; 24(7):386–91. Stein DG.

Estrogen protects against injury from epilepsy. Neuroscientist. 2007 Feb; 13(1):77–88. Veliskova J.

Estrogen deficiency is associated with age-related hearing loss. Amer J Ob/Gyn 2004 Jan; 190(1):77–82. Kilicdag EB et al.

Estrogen increases BDNF. Front Neuro Endocrinol. 2006 Oct 19; Scharfman HE et al.

Estrogen protects against Alzheimer's disease. Adv Etp Meg Bio 1997; 429:261–71. Chang D et al.; Menopause 2006 Jul-Aug; 13(4):584–91. Boccardi M et al. Neurology 57:605–612. Asthana S et al. Proc Natl Acad Sci USA 2005. 102:19198–19203.

Estrogen regulates functions of RPE (Retinal Pigment Epithelium) and its deficiency during menopause period may be a factor contributing to the development of age-related macular degeneration in elderly women. Mech Ageing Dev 2005 Nov;126(11):1135–45. Yu X et al .

We discuss the protective effects of the sex hormones, estradiol, progesterone and testosterone with a specific focus on mitochondrial dysfunction in AD. Neurosci Bio Behav Rev 2016 Aug; 67:89–101. Grimm A et al.

Estrogen receptor β deficiency impairs BDNF-signaling in the hippocampus of female brain. A possible mechanism for menopausal depression. Psychoneuroendocrinology 2017 Aug; 82:107–116. Chhibber A et al.

The loss of functional ERα may lead to deregulation of post ischemic inflammatory responses and increased vulnerability to ischemic injury in aging female brains. Neurobiol Aging 2016 Apr; 40:50–60. Cordeau P et al.

BONE AND MUSCLE

Bioidentical estradiol promotes muscle growth and regeneration. J Appl Physiol 2006 Jun; 100(6):2012–23. McClung JM et al.

Significant increase of osteoporosis and bone fracture in women who stop taking estrogen. Climacteric 2007 Aug; 10(4):273–5. Gambaccini M et al.

Declines in endogenous estrogen levels after menopause can lead to systemic bone loss, including loss of oral bone. J Periodontol 2015 Apr; 86(4):595–605. Wang Y et al.

Current data provide evidence about the beneficial effect of vitamin D supplementation on muscle strength, physical performance and prevention of falls and fractures in elderly female populations. Maturitas 2015 Sep; 82(1):56–64. Anagnostis P et al.

MITOCHONDRIA

Estrogen control mitochondrial function and biogenesis. Cell Biochem 2008 Dec; 105(6):1342–51. Kline CM et al.

E2 promotes the energetic capacity of brain mitochondria by maximizing aerobic glycolysis (preventing AD) Adv Drug Deliv Rev 2008 Oct-Nov; 30(13-14): 1504–11. Brinton RD et al.

Estrogen prevents cell death by maintaining functionally intact mitochondria. Brain Res Rev 2008 Mar; 57(2):421–30. Simpkins JW et al.

Estrogen: An emerging regulator of insulin action and mitochondrial function. J Diabetes Res 2015; 2015:916585. Gupte AA et al.

ESTROGEN AND WEIGHT LOSS

Prolonged estradiol treatment increases insulin sensitivity. Mol Endocrinol 2006 Jun; 20(6):1287–99. Gao H et al.

Prevention of obesity and insulin resistance by estrogens. Diabetes 2013; July 31. Handgraaf S et al.

Bioidentical estradiol decreases body fat. Philos Trans R Soc Lond B Biol Sci 2006 Jul 29; 361(1471):1251–63. Asarian L et al.

Estradiol helps overcome leptin resistance in mice on high fat diet. Horm Metab Res 2010 Mar; 42(3):182–6. Matyskova R et al.

Bioidentical estradiol applied to skin decreases ghrelin. Fertil Steril 2006 Dec; 86(6) 1669. Micheline CC et al.

Bioidentical estradiol increases CCK, satiety, and decreases food intake. Philos Trans R Soc Lond B Biol Sci 2006 Jul 29; 361(1471):1251–63. Asarian L et al.

Decline of estrogen leads to binge-eating. Psychol Med 2006 Oct 12; 1–11. Edler C et al.

Estrogen replacement therapy can improve insulin resistance by lowering body weight. In addition, it can exert its effect directly on adipose tissue, improve the levels of adipokines, reduce the amount of visceral fat, and improve insulin sensitivity in mice. Zhongguo Yi Xue Ke Xue Yuan Xue Bao 2015 Jun; 37(3):269–73. Yuan T et al.

Bioidentical estradiol cream is more effective in managing weight and insulin sensitivity than capsule form. Fertil Steril 2006 Dec; 86(6)1669. Micheline CC et al.

Estrogen deficiency causes increase in appetite and reduces energy expenditure, promoting weight gain and ultimately causing obesity. Best Pract Res Clin Endocrinol Metab 2016 Aug; 30(4):527–536. Lopez M et al.

E beta receptor increases energy expenditure and brown adipose tissue. FASEB J 2016 Oct 12. Ponnsamy S et al.

Menopausal hormone therapy is associated with reduced total and visceral adiposity. J Clin Endocrinol Metab 2018 May 1; 103(5):1948–1957. Papadakis GE et al.

GENERAL

The association between vulvar pain and bladder pain is related to a vaginal environment carrying signs of hypoestrogenism. Gynecol Endocrinol 2015 Oct; 31(10):828–32. Gardella B et al.

Hormone replacement, as reported here, could possibly slow the loss of alveoli due to the aging process. Anat Rec (Hoboken) 2016 Apr 16. Herring MJ et al.

New-onset asthma and respiratory symptoms increased in women becoming postmenopausal. Allergy Clin Immunol 2016 Jan; 137(1):50–57.e6. Triebner K et al.

Duration of estrogen deficiency in post-menopausal state confers fibrosis risk among post-menopausal women with NAFLD. Hepatology 2016 Feb 26. Klair JS et al.

In the ovariectomized female rats model, exogenous estrogen can significantly up-regulate telomerase activity and TERT mRNA expression to exert the effects of anti-aging. Gynecol Endocrinol 2015 Jul; 31(7):582–5. Cen J et al.

A longer leukocyte telomere length (LTL) in women than men has been attributed to a slow rate of LTL attrition in women, perhaps due to high estrogen exposure during the premenopausal period. Int J Epidemiol 2015 Oct; 44(5):1688–95. Dalgård C et al.

KRAS-VARIANT

Estrogen withdrawal and a low estrogen state appear to increase BC risk and to predict aggressive tumor biology in women with the KRAS-variant, who are also significantly more likely to present with multiple primary breast cancer. Cell Cycle 2015; 14(13):2091–9. McVeigh TP et al.

AROMATASE INHIBITOR ASSOCIATED MUSCULOSKELETAL SYNDROME (AIMSS)

Estrogen deprivation leads to incapacitating AIMSS. Steroid 2011 Jul; 76(8):781–5. Lintermans A et al.

AIMSS occurs in approximately 50% of AI treated patients. Br J Cancer 2010 July; 103(3):291–6. Henry NC et al.

Widespread body pain increased the risk of cancer and reduced cancer survival. Arthritis Rheum 2003 Jun; 48(6):1686–92. McBeth J et al.

Opioids are used to treat AIMSS. Breast Cancer Research 2011; 13:205. Gaillard S and Stearns V.

Opioids impair immunity response, increase angiogenesis, and encourage tumor cells to grow and spread. Anesthesiology 2012 Apr; 116(4): 940–5. Moss J et al.

Anti-estrogenic endocrine therapy decreases EVL (EVL may be implicated in invasion and/or metastasis of human breast cancer). Nat Commun 2018 Jul 30; 9(1):2980. Parker SS et al.

BREAST CANCER—SAFETY OF ESTROGEN WITH AND WITHOUT BREAST CANCER

Hormone replacement therapy in women with a history of breast cancer. Gynecol Endocrinol 2002 Dec; 16(6):469–78. Ylikorkala O et al.; Int J Fertil Womens Med 1999 Jun-Aug; 44(4):186–92. Brewster WR et al.

Effects of estrogens and hormone replacement therapy on breast cancer risk and on efficacy of breast cancer therapies. Maturitas 2000 Jul 31; 36(1):1–17. Verheul HA et al.

HRT in postmenopausal women yields decrease in cancer aggression . . . metastasis free and global survival were better in the HRT group. Bull Cancer 2007 May; 94(5):469–75. Czernichow C et al.

GENERAL

More than 1.5 servings of red meat a day increases risk of breast cancer by 97%. Arch Intern Med 2006 Nov 13; 166(20): 2253–9. Cho E et al.

High versus low intake of smoked beef/lamb/pork was associated with a 17% increased hazard of all-cause and a 23% increased hazard of breast cancer–specific mortality. J Natl Cancer Inst 2017 109 (6). Parada H et al.

Antibiotic treatment significantly increases risk for breast cancer. 51–100 days of meds increase by 53%. 501–1000 days of use increase incidence by 114%. JAMA 2004; 291(7): 827–35. Velicer C et al.

Gain of more than 22 pounds since menopause increases risk of breast cancer by 18%. JAMA 2006; 296: 193–201. Eliassen AH et al.

Weight gain and weight cycling were positively associated with risk of breast (11%) and endometrial cancer (23%), respectively. Cancer Epidemiol Biomarkers Prev 2017 Jan 9. Welti LM et al.

Postmenopausal women with adolescent leanness were only associated with increased breast cancer risk when excess weight was gained during adulthood (52% increase). Cancer Epidemiol 2016 Dec; 45:135–144. Florath I et al.

Weight gain since age eighteen was positively associated with ER+/PR+ postmenopausal breast cancer (50% increase). Int J Cancer 2017 Jan 30. Rosner B et al.

Weight gain in perimenopause decreases breast cancer. JAMA Oncol 2018 Jan 21: E181771. Sander OP et al.

Current smoker has 16% increase in breast cancer. BMJ 2011 Mar; 342:d1016. Margolis K et al.

Passive smoking for twenty years increased breast cancer by 27%; smoking over twenty years increased BC by 264%. PLoS One 2017 Feb 2; 12(2):e0171198. Strumylaite L et al.

Current smokers have a higher breast-cancer-specific mortality of 30% and higher all-cause mortality of 52%. Breast 2017 Mar 31; 33:117–124. Duan W et al.

Consumption of bad fat (Omega 6) increases risk of breast cancer by more than 100%. Cancer Causes Control 2002 Dec; 13(10): 883–93. Wirfalt E et al.

Grismaijer et al. examined the 4,700 bra-wearing US women. Three out of four women who wore their bras twenty-four hours per day developed breast cancer. One out of seven women who wore bras more than twelve hours per day (but not to bed) developed breast cancer. One out of 168 women who wore bras rarely or never acquired breast cancer. *Dressed to Kill* 2002. Grismaijer S et al.

Grapefruit intake may increase the risk of breast cancer among postmenopausal women by 30%. Br J Cancer 2007 Aug; 97(3):440–5. Monroe KR et al.

Studies on the association between the use of calcium channel blockers (CCBs) and breast cancer risk. PLoS One 2014 Sep 3; 9(9):e105801. Li W et al.

ACE (angiotensin-converting enzyme inhibitors) exposure was associated with BC recurrence of 56%. Breast Cancer Res Treat 2011 Sep; 129(2):549–56. Ganz PA et al.

Long-term exposure to dietary sources of genistein induces estrogen-independence in the human breast cancer (MCF-7) xenograft model with more aggressive and advanced growth phenotypes. Mol Nutr Food Res 2014 Feb 24. Andrade JE et al.

Lifetime genistein intake increases the response of mammary tumors to tamoxifen in rats. Clin Cancer Res 2017 Feb 1; 23(3):814–824. Zhang X et al.

The effects of combinatorial genistein and sulforaphane in breast tumor inhibition. Int J Mol Sci 2018 Jun 13; 19(6). Paul B et al.

Current digoxin users were at increased risk of BC by 45%. Risk normalized when digoxin was stopped. J Clin Oncol 2011 Jun 1; 29(16):2165–70. Biggar RJ et al.

Black cohosh increases metastatic mammary cancer in transgenic mice expressing c-erbB2. Cancer Res 2008 Oct 15; 68(20):8377–83. Davis VL et al.

Obese women who used hydrophobic statins (simvastatin) had an elevated risk of progesterone receptor-negative breast cancer (400%). Anticancer Res 2009 Dec; 29(12): 5143–8. Eaton M et al.

Risk of breast cancer increases by 210% from taking birth control before the age of twenty. Eur J Cancer 2005; 41(15): 2312–20. Jernstrom H et al.

Birth control significantly increases incidence of breast cancer, if started at young age, and lasted over twelve years (40%). Breast Cancer Res Treat 1998 Jul; 50(2):175–84. Ursin G et al.

Increased risk of breast cancer by 30% with long duration of oral contraceptive. J Natl Cancer Inst 1994 Apr 6; 86(7):505–14. White E et al.

Recent oral contraceptive use (within the prior year) was associated with an increased breast cancer risk 50%, relative to never using or formerly using OC. The association was stronger for estrogen receptor-positive (70%). Cancer Res 2014 Aug 1; 74(15):4078–89. Beaber EF et al.

Women who are less active have 16% increase in breast cancer. Active women have 10% reduction of invasive breast cancer. Cancer Epidemiology Biomarkers Prev 2014 Sep; 23(9):1893–902. Fournier A et al.

Lack of physical activity is associated with shortened TL (telomere length). Breast Cancer Res 2014 Jul 31; 16(4): 413. Garland SN et al.

Among postmenopausal women, physical activity decreased the chance of developing breast cancer by 49%. Biomed Res Int 2018 Jul 12. Mota JF et al.

Adherence to the Western dietary pattern was related to higher risk of breast cancer up to 46%; especially in premenopausal women the increase was 75%. In contrast, the Mediterranean pattern was related to a lower risk and decrease of 44% in breast cancer. Br J Cancer 2014 Sep 23; 111(7):1454–62. Castello A et al.

Metabolic syndrome increases the death from breast cancer by 23% for women over 60. Cancer Epidemiol Biomarkers Prev 2010 Jul; 19(7):1737–45. Bjorge T et al.

Insulin resistance showed statistically significant association to HER-2+ (increase 210%) and luminal breast tumors. Diabetol Metab Syndr 2014 Sep 26; 6(1):105. Capasso L et al.

MS (metabolic syndrome) was associated with a 52% increase in cancer risk. Menopause 2013 Dec; 20(12):1301–9. Esposito K et al.

Multicenter study conducted in Italy and Switzerland on 3,869 cases of breast cancer in postmenopause reported a relative risk of 1.75 in women with the metabolic syndrome. Recenti Prog Med 2011 Dec; 102(12):476–8. Rosato V et al.

People with lactose intolerance, characterized by low consumption of milk and other dairy products, had decreased risks of breast cancer by 21%. Br J Cancer 2014 Oct 14. Ji J et al.

A significant twofold increased risk of breast cancer among premenopausal and postmenopausal women was observed in the highest quartile of sugar intake. A higher intake of dietary fiber was associated with a significantly lower breast cancer risk among both premenopausal (69%) and postmenopausal (73%) women. Asian Pac J Cancer Prev 2014; 15(14):5959–64. Sulaiman S et al.

Breast cancer for the highest versus the lowest quintile was 28% higher for bread. Ann Oncol 2013 Dec; 24(12):3094–9. Augustin LS et al.

Women in the highest glucose quartile had a significantly greater risk of breast cancer (63%) than those in the lowest glucose quartile. Int J Cancer 2012 Feb 15; 130(4):921–9. Sieri S et al.

Consumption of dessert foods was associated with a 55% increase in breast cancer. Cancer Causes Control 2009 Oct; 20(8):1509–15. Bradshaw PT et al.

Compared with women with the lowest tertile of intake, women in the highest tertile of intake of desserts had 19% increase in breast cancer. Ann Oncol 2006 Feb; 17(2):341–5. Tavani A et al.

"Significant trends across categories of alcohol consumption were observed, with hazard ratios for those consuming 7 or more drinks per week versus never drinkers as follows: for estrogen receptor-positive (ER+) cancer, 48% increase, for progesterone receptor-positive 64% increase, for ER+/PR+ cancer 63% increase, and for mixed ductal/lobular cancer 250% increase." Am J Epidemiology 2014 Oct 1; 180(7):705–17. Falk RT et al.

Breast cancer screening was not associated with a reduction in the incidence of advanced cancer. It is likely that 1 in every 3 invasive tumors and cases of DCIS diagnosed in women offered screening represent overdiagnosis (incidence increase of 48.3%). Ann Intern Med 2017 Jan 10. Jørgensen KJ et al.

Detection and treatment of low-grade DCIS and invasive tubular cancer would appear to represent overdiagnosis in most cases. Breast 2016 Oct 28. Evans A et al.

Authorities acknowledge that screening mammogram harms include 30% increase in overdiagnosis and overtreatment, delayed diagnosis, and radiation-induced cancer. Only 7% of the patients are given this information before the screening mammogram. Health Expect 2008; 11:366–375. Nekhlyudov L et al.

The repeat mammographic group has had 22% more breast cancer. Arch Int Med 2008 Nov; 168(21):2311–6. Welch HG et al.

Repeated screening starting at age 50 saves about 1.8 lives over 15 years for every 1,000 women screened. The number needed to screen repeatedly is 1000/1.8, or 556. The survival percentage is 99.12% without and 99.29% with screening. BMC Med Inform Decis Mak 2009 Apr 2; 9:18. Keen JD.

WHI STUDY—WHAT A MESS

Trudy Bush, MD, summarized 25 years and 50 reports on HRT and ERT and concluded that estrogen treatment is no risk factor for increased breast cancer. This study was published in 2001. Obstet and Gynecol 2001 Sep; 98(3): 498–508. Bush TL et al.

The WHI study was conducted on women who were 10–20 years into menopause with HRT. JAMA 2002 Jul 17; 288(3): 321–33. Rossouw JE et al.

The public failed to hear that in the WHI study's use of Premarin alone, there was a 23% decrease in breast cancer. JAMA 2013 Oct; 310(13):1353–68. Manson JE et al.

Over a 10-year span, starting in 2002, at least 18,601 and as many as 91,610 postmenopausal women died prematurely because of the avoidance of estrogen therapy. In younger postmenopausal women estrogen therapy is associated with a decisive reduction in all-cause mortality, but estrogen use in this population is low and continuing to fall. Am J Public Health 2013 Sep; 103(9): 1583–93. Sarrel PM et al.

Holly Thacker, MD, is the director of the Center for Specialized Women's Health at the Cleveland Clinic in Cleveland, Ohio, and Professor of Obstetrics and Gynecology and Women's Health. Extended WHI follow-up: a reduction in all-cause mortality among women who initiated HT within 10 years of menopause, whether they used estrogen alone (women with hysterectomies) or estrogen-progestin therapy (women with an intact uterus), compared with women in the placebo group. JAMA 2013; 310(13):1353–1368. Manson JE et al.

"After the WHI trial was published in 2003, use of HT dropped 70% within 5 years in Norway and Sweden while breast cancer rates were essentially unchanged. After 2008, HT use has dropped further and breast cancer incidence rates have started increasing again. The study objective is to calculate and to explain potential bias in the observational study design. Here we use data from the randomized WHI trial and analyze these data as done in the observational studies to calculate the magnitude of the potential biases in the observational study design. Other risk factors for the increase in breast cancer risk in the age group 50–69 years should be considered, for example, over diagnosis. In simplicity, the statistic that WHI used was false." PLoS One 2015 May 4; 10(5):e0124076. Zahl PH et al.

"Obtained cumulative hazard plots, hazard ratios, and outcome rates from the simulated model did not show differences in relation to the original WHI report. The differences in RMST (restricted mean survival time) between placebo and conjugated equine estrogens 0.625 mg plus medroxyprogesterone acetate 2.5 mg (in flexible parametric modeling) were 1.17 days, (95% CI, −2.25 to 4.59) for invasive breast cancer, 7.50 days (95% CI, 2.90 to 12.11) for coronary heart disease, 2.75 days (95% CI, −0.84 to 6.34) for stroke, 4.23 days (95% CI, 1.82 to 6.64) for pulmonary embolism, −2.73 days (95% CI, −5.32 to −0.13) for colorectal cancer, and −2.77 days (95% CI, −5.44 to −0.1) for hip fracture. Conclusions: The differences in RMST for the outcomes of the WHI study are too small to establish clinical risks related to hormone therapy use." Menopause 2015 May 11. Aedo S et al.

"Subsequent reanalyses of data from the WHI with age stratification, newer randomized and observational data and several meta-analyses now consistently show reductions in CHD and mortality when HRT is initiated soon after menopause. HRT also significantly decreases the incidence of various symptoms of menopause and the risk of osteoporotic fractures, and improves quality of life." Nat Rev Endocrinol 2016 Oct 7. Lobo RA et al.

With the "alarming initial WHI report... HRT use plummeted world-wide, driven by fear of breast cancer and skepticism about cardiovascular benefits. Stunningly, the contrasting findings of the WHI trial of CEE alone reported 2 years later—suggesting prevention of coronary heart disease in women who began HRT at age <60 years, and a reduction in breast cancer overall—were largely ignored. . . . Critically, the 'facts' that most women and clinicians consider in making the decision to use, or not use, HRT are frequently wrong or incorrectly applied." Climacteric 2017 Apr; 20(2):91–96. Langer RD.

"However, perhaps the most egregious part . . ." *Estrogen Matters: Why Taking Hormones in Menopause Can Improve Women's Well-Being and Lengthen Their Lives—Without Raising the Risk of Breast Cancer*, Avrum Bluming, M.D., and Carol Tavris, Ph.D. (Little Brown, 2018). Bluming and Tavris cite: Risks and benefits of hormone therapy: Has medical dogma now been overturned? Climacteric 2014; 17:215–22. Shapiro S., de Villers TJ, Pines A et al.; Risks of estrogen plus progestin therapy: A sensitivity analysis of the findings in the Women's Health Initiative randomizes controlled trial. Climacteric 2003; 6:302–10. Shapiro, S.

HOW ESTROGEN PROTECTS BREASTS

Estrogen increases apoptosis. J Steroid Biochem Mol Biol 2000; 72(3-4): 89–102. Szelei J et al.; Menopause 2013 Apr; 20(4):372–82. Jordan VC et al.

Estradiol reduces NFKbeta, IL 6, and IL 11. J Huazhong Univ Sci Technology Med Sci 2006; 26(1): 53–8. Wang Y et al.

Estrogen decreases breast cancer stem cell. Breast Can Res and Treat 2011 Aug; 129(1):23–35. Simoes BM et al.

Estrogen deprivation reduced (while estradiol increased) p53 levels. Cancer Res Treat 2011 Jan; 125(1):35–42. Fernandez-Cuesta L et al.

Expression of proinflammatory mediators Cox-2, TNFα, IL1β and aromatase was reduced in the mammary glands of mice that received supplemental E2. This was achieved via ER alpha. Cancer Prev Res Aug 2015; 8(8):751–9. Bhardwaj P et al.

ESTROGEN AS BREAST CANCER TREATMENT

Estrogen was the standard of care treatment for postmenopausal women with metastatic breast cancer. Br Med J 1944; 2:3938. Haddow A et al.

In 1970 tamoxifen was introduced. When both were compared (tamoxifen/DES), the responses were equivalent, yet tamoxifen has fewer immediate side effects. New England J Med 1981; 304:16–21. Ingle JN et al.

Physiological data and clinical outcomes demonstrate that bioidentical hormones are associated with lower risks, including the risk of breast cancer and cardiovascular disease, and are more efficacious than their synthetic and animal-derived counterparts. Until evidence is found to the contrary, bioidentical hormones remain the preferred method of HRT. Further randomized controlled trials are needed to delineate these differences more clearly. Postgrad Med 2009 Jan; 121(1):73–85. Holtorf K.

When the antiestrogen treatment fails or gets to be resistant, the treatment is a high dose of estrogen. Breast 2005 Dec; 14(6):624–30. Jordan VC et al.; World J Surg Oncol 2006 Jul 11; 4: 44. Agrawal A et al.; Med Ped Oncol 1990; 18: 317–20. Boyer MJ et al.; JAMA 2009; 302:774–80. Ellis JM et al.; Br J of Cancer 2013 Sep; 109(6):1537–42. Iwase H et al.

"Our data suggest, with respect to tamoxifen, that its use as a chemopreventant in women at high risk of developing breast cancer (Kiang 1991) should be viewed with caution, since in the presence of tamoxifen, subpopulations of cells may arise that are stimulated, rather than inhibited, by the drug." J Natl Cancer Inst 1991 Apr 3; 83(7):462–3. Kiang DT.

ERT after breast cancer treatment does not seem to increase a breast cancer event. J Clin Oncol 1999 May; 17(5): 1482–7. Vassilopoulou-Sellin R et al.

Followup of women with breast cancer on HRT shows no increase of breast cancer death or recurrence. Arch Family Med 1966 Jun; 5(6):341–8. Gambreal RD; Am J OB/GYN 1996 May; 174(5):1494–8. Disaia PJ et al.

The risks of recurrence and mortality are lower in women who used HRT after breast cancer diagnosis than in women who did not. J Natl Cancer Inst 2001 May; 93(10):754–62. O'Meara ES et al.

Menopausal HT use in breast cancer survivors was not associated with increased cancer recurrence, cancer-related mortality, or total mortality. Maturitas 2006 Jan 20; 53(2):123–32. Batur P et al.

The refusal to give HRT to women with breast cancer "is not . . . supported by the observational data . . . because HRT has not increased the risk for breast cancer recurrence." Gynecol Endocrinol 2002 Dec; 16(6):469–78. Ylikorkala O et al.

The concern that ERT might activate growth in occult metastatic sites and promote a rash of recurrences was not confirmed. Med. 1999 Jun-Aug; 44(4):186–92. Brewster WR et al.

"The study group consisted of 123 women (mean age, 65.4 +/– 8.85 years) who were diagnosed with breast cancer in our practice, including 69 patients who received estrogen replacement therapy for > or = 32 years after diagnosis. Estrogen replacement therapy apparently does not increase either the risk of recurrence or of death in patients with early breast cancer." Am J Obstet Gynecol 2002 Aug; 187(2):289–94; discussion 294–5. Natarajan PK et al.

Hormone replacement therapy in breast cancer survivors: a cohort study. "No obvious adverse effect of hormone replacement therapy could be shown in this pilot study." Am J Obstet Gynecol 1996 May; 174(5):1494–8. Disaia PJ.

Hormone therapy for women after breast cancer revealed no increase in recurrent disease among treated patients. J Reprod Med 2004 Jul; 49(7):510–26. Levgur M.

Use of ERT in a cohort of breast cancer survivors with tumors of generally good prognosis was not associated with increased breast cancer events compared with non-ERT users, even over a long followup period. Ann Surg Oncol 2001 Dec; 8(10):828–32. Peters GN et al.

Studies have shown no adverse effects of an estrogen or an estrogen-progestin replacement therapy after treatment of a mammary carcinoma. Anticancer Res 1998 May-Jun; 18(3C):2253–5. Braendle W.

No association was found between HRT use and risk of BC recurrence. Breast 2018 40:123–130. Wang Y et al.

Agreement to give HRT to women with BC. Crit Rev Oncol Hematol 2018; 124:51–60. Gatti et al.

Reduced incidence of distant metastases and lower mortality in 1,072 patients with breast cancer with a history of hormone replacement therapy. Am J Obstet Gynecol 2007 Apr; 196(4):342.e1–9. Schuetz F et al.

No increase of fatal breast cancer with HRT. Pharmacoepidemiol Drug Saf 2010 May; 19(5):440–447. Norman SA et al.

There seems to be little if any risk in giving hormone replacement therapy to women who have had breast or endometrial cancer. There is no data to suggest that hormone replacement therapy is contraindicated in women who have been treated for cervical or ovarian cancer. Curr Opin Oncol 2005 Sep; 17(5):493–9. Creastman WT.

ERT to 277 stable breast cancer patients, shown no increase in recurrence or death. Menopause 2003 Jul-Aug; 10(4):277–85. Decker DA et al.

When used alone, CEE are not associated with an increased risk of breast cancer and may be associated with reduced mortality. Expert Opin Drug Saf 2014 Jan; 13(1):45–56. Mirkin S et al.

Two Sister Study: 1,419 cases diagnosed with breast cancer before the age of 50 years and 1,665 controls. Estrogen alone showed 42% reduction of BC. American J Epidemiology 2015; 181(10):799–807. O'Brien KM et al.

HRT AND BREAST CANCER RISK

Followup information was obtained on 3,303 women with a median duration of followup of 17 years. The relative risk (RR) of developing breast cancer was 0.98 for women who took exogenous estrogens as compared to 1.8 for women who did not. Exogenous estrogens lowered the observed breast cancer risk in women with atypical hyperplasia (RR=3.0 versus 4.5). Cancer 1989 Mar 1; 63(5):948. Dupont WD et al.

Estradiol-only therapy carries no risk for breast cancer, estradiol therapy combined with dydrogesterone and progesterone carries no risk of breast cancer. Gynecol Endocrinol 2017 Feb; 33(2):87–92. Yang Z et al.

HRT in postmenopausal women yields decrease in cancer aggression. Metastasis free and global survival were better in the HRT group l. Bull Cancer 2007 NAY; 94(5):469–75. This P et al.

HRT in menopause does not affect increase of risk of death of any form. J Clin Endo Meta 2015; 100(11):4021–8. Murad MH et al.

BC increased 48% with use of hormonal IUD in postmenopausal women. Cancer Causes Control 2016; 27(2):249–58. Sarkeala T et al.

These facts support no significant effect of HRT history in the risk of breast cancer in Korean women. J Prev Med Public Health 2015 Sep; 48(5):225–30. Bae JM, Kim EH.

HRT after oophorectomy to BRCA1 carriers—no increase of BC. JAMA Oncol 2018; (8):1059–1065. Karlan BY et al.

Incidence of BC in a 22-year study with estrogen-progestin replacement therapy: initial 10 years, BC in the placebo group was 4.8%, no cancers were found in the hormone replacement therapy group. After an additional 12 years of followup, the overall incidence of breast cancer in the women who had never taken hormone replacement therapy was 11.5%. No breast cancers had developed in the women who were on HRT. Obstet Gynecol 1992 Nov; 80(5):827–30. Nachtigall MJ et al.

Between 2010 and 2015 3% of women with BC on AI or tamoxifen used bioidentical HRT. Obstet Gynecol 2018 Oct 5. Huntley JH et al.

The use of estrogen with progestin HRT does not appear to be associated with an increased risk of breast cancer in middle-aged (50 to 64 years) women, including 537 patients with incident primary breast cancer diagnosed between January 1, 1988, and June 30, 1990. JAMA 1995 Jul 12; 274(2):137–42. Stanford J et al.

"Ever-use of ERT was associated with a significantly decreased risk of fatal breast cancer by 16%. There was a moderate trend (P = 0.07) of decreasing risk with younger age at first use of ERT. This decreased risk was most pronounced in women who experienced natural menopause before the age of 40 years." Cancer Causes Control 1996 Jul; 7(4):449–57. Willis DB et al.

HRT was associated with a decrease in breast cancer in BRCA1 population. J Natl Cancer Inst 2008 Oct 1; 100(19):1361–7. Eisen A et al.

French study of bioidentical estradiol and progesterone showed decreased breast cancer in users compared to nonusers. Gynecol Endocrinol 2006 Aug; 22(8): 423–31. Espie M et al.

Harvard University study of use of Premarin alone shows no increase of incidence of breast cancer for 15 years. Cancer Epidemiology Biomarkers Prev 2006 Jan; 15(1):39–44. Gann P et al.

A study of 9,000 Japanese women found HRT users less likely to develop breast cancer than never users. Proc ASCO 2006; 24:10012. Takeuchi M et al.

Bio HRT treatment decreased the risk of breast cancer. J Clinic Oncol 2009 Nov; 27(31):5138–43. Fournier A et al.

Reduced risk of death from BC in HRT users compared with nonusers. Amer J Obst Gynecol 2002 Feb; 186(2):325–34. Nanda K et al.

PREGNANCY PROTECTS THE BREAST

Pregnancy after breast cancer significantly increases survival (up to 50%) and decreases cancer recurrence and metastasis, compared to breast cancer survivors who did not get pregnant; multiple studies confirm this observation. BMJ 2007 Jan 27; 334(7586):194. Ives A et al.; Cancer 2003 Sep 15; 98(6):1131–40. Mueller BA et al.; Laeknabladid 2000 July/August; 86(7/8):495–498. Birgisson H et al.; Cancer 1999 Jun 1; 85(11):2424–32. Velentgas P et al.; Ob Gyn Surv 2010 Dec; 65(12):786–793. Valachis A et al.; Cancer 2009 Nov 15; 115(22):5155–65. Largillier R et al.

"At a median follow-up of 7.2 years after pregnancy, no difference in disease-free survival was observed between pregnant and nonpregnant patients with ER-positive . . . or ER-negative disease . . . [P]atients in the pregnant cohort had better O[verall] S[urvival]" (43%). J National Cancer Institute 2018; 110(4):426–29. Ameye L et al.

High level of estriol in one pregnancy decreased the overall risk of breast cancer by 58%. The U.S. Army Medical Research and Materiel Command DAMD17-99-1-9358. Pentii K et al.

A Norwegian study with 63,090 women observed "strong and highly significant inverse association between the number of full-term pregnancies and the risk of breast cancer." Eur J Cancer 1992; 28a(6-7):1148–53. Vatten LJ et al.

Breast cancer risk drops with each pregnancy by 7%. Lancet 2002 Jul 20; 360(9328): 187–95. Collaborative Group on Hormonal Factors in Breast Cancer.

Teenage pregnancy associated with decreased risk of breast cancer. Int J Food Sci and Nutr 1995 Nov; 46(4):373–81. Walker AR et al.

Nulliparity was associated with increased risk for all breast cancers. Cancer 2011 May; 117(9):1946–1956. Newcomb PA et al.

Early full-term pregnancy has been shown to reduce the lifetime risk of breast cancer. Prog Mol Biol Transl Sci 2017; 151:81–111. Subramani R et al.

Acknowledgments

Writing a book while still working full-time as a physician can only happen with the greatest team around me. I would like to thank Billie Fitzpatrick, who, as my co-writer and researcher, also inspired me; my agent, Peter McGuigan of Foundry Literary & Media, and others at Foundry who were instrumental in matching me with the perfect publishing house; and thanks also to my publishing team at St. Martin's Press, including my editor extraordinaire, Elizabeth Beier, and her right-hand editorial assistant, Hannah Phillips, who understood the vision of my book and brought it to fruition.

Index